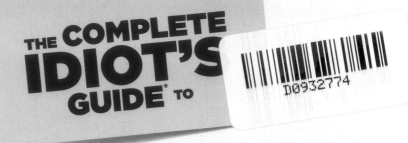

THE COMPLETE IDIOT'S GUIDE TO

Low-Sodium Cooking

Second Edition

by Shelly Vaughan James and Heidi McIndoo, R.D.

ILLINOIS PRAIRIE DISTRICT LIBRARY

A

A member of Per

ILLINOIS PRAIRIE DPL

A65502 121576

641.5
JAM

To my young writer and illustrator, keep your dream alive always. —Shelly

To my husband Sean, for always supporting me through all the highs and lows of trying to combine nutrition and writing into a successful career while at the same time being a full-time mom and wife. —Heidi

ALPHA BOOKS

Published by the Penguin Group

Penguin Group (USA) Inc., 375 Hudson Street, New York, New York 10014, USA

Penguin Group (Canada), 90 Eglinton Avenue East, Suite 700, Toronto, Ontario M4P 2Y3, Canada (a division of Pearson Penguin Canada Inc.)

Penguin Books Ltd., 80 Strand, London WC2R 0RL, England

Penguin Ireland, 25 St. Stephen's Green, Dublin 2, Ireland (a division of Penguin Books Ltd.)

Penguin Group (Australia), 250 Camberwell Road, Camberwell, Victoria 3124, Australia (a division of Pearson Australia Group Pty. Ltd.)

Penguin Books India Pvt. Ltd., 11 Community Centre, Panchsheel Park, New Delhi—110 017, India

Penguin Group (NZ), 67 Apollo Drive, Rosedale, North Shore, Auckland 1311, New Zealand (a division of Pearson New Zealand Ltd.)

Penguin Books (South Africa) (Pty.) Ltd., 24 Sturdee Avenue, Rosebank, Johannesburg 2196, South Africa

Penguin Books Ltd., Registered Offices: 80 Strand, London WC2R 0RL, England

First edition originally published as *The Complete Idiot's Guide to Low-Sodium Meals*

Copyright © 2011 by Shelly Vaughan James

All rights reserved. No part of this book shall be reproduced, stored in a retrieval system, or transmitted by any means, electronic, mechanical, photocopying, recording, or otherwise, without written permission from the publisher. No patent liability is assumed with respect to the use of the information contained herein. Although every precaution has been taken in the preparation of this book, the publisher and authors assume no responsibility for errors or omissions. Neither is any liability assumed for damages resulting from the use of information contained herein. For information, address Alpha Books, 800 East 96th Street, Indianapolis, IN 46240.

THE COMPLETE IDIOT'S GUIDE TO and Design are registered trademarks of Penguin Group (USA) Inc.

International Standard Book Number: 978-1-61564-132-1
Library of Congress Catalog Card Number: 2011908143

13 12 11   8 7 6 5 4 3 2 1

Interpretation of the printing code: The rightmost number of the first series of numbers is the year of the book's printing; the rightmost number of the second series of numbers is the number of the book's printing. For example, a printing code of 11-1 shows that the first printing occurred in 2011.

Printed in the United States of America

Note: This publication contains the opinions and ideas of its authors. It is intended to provide helpful and informative material on the subject matter covered. It is sold with the understanding that the authors and publisher are not engaged in rendering professional services in the book. If the reader requires personal assistance or advice, a competent professional should be consulted.

The authors and publisher specifically disclaim any responsibility for any liability, loss, or risk, personal or otherwise, which is incurred as a consequence, directly or indirectly, of the use and application of any of the contents of this book.

Most Alpha books are available at special quantity discounts for bulk purchases for sales promotions, premiums, fund-raising, or educational use. Special books, or book excerpts, can also be created to fit specific needs.

For details, write: Special Markets, Alpha Books, 375 Hudson Street, New York, NY 10014.

Publisher: *Marie Butler-Knight*
Associate Publisher/Acquiring Editor: *Mike Sanders*
Executive Managing Editor: *Billy Fields*
Senior Development Editor: *Christy Wagner*
Senior Production Editor: *Kayla Dugger*
Copy Editor: *Monica Stone*

Cover Designer: *Kurt Owens*
Book Designers: *William Thomas, Rebecca Batchelor*
Indexer: *Julie Bess*
Layout: *Ayanna Lacey*
Senior Proofreader: *Laura Caddell*

Contents

Introduction

When you picked up this cookbook, you probably hoped for a few delicious recipes you could prepare knowing that the meals complemented your lower sodium needs. Naturally, we've included hundreds of mouthwatering recipes, all of them low in sodium. But we believe the best test of a great cookbook is if you, the reader, can take away what you've learned and put into practice the measures and methods you need to live a more healthful life.

Sodium has received a lot of attention since we first published this book 5 years ago. Additional studies and increased research have resulted in even lower sodium recommendation guidelines for even healthy adults. Fortunately, food manufacturers and retailers have taken note, reducing the sodium in commercial offerings, while restaurants are making better choices available to health-conscious consumers.

Still, you may be standing in your kitchen empty-handed where your salt shaker or other sodium-laden seasonings once firmly rested. If you're facing eating constraints that aren't entirely clear to you, we're here to help. Beyond the more than 300 flavorful, taste-bud-intriguing recipes in this book, we've also shared the information you need to know for cooking in a sodium-sensible kitchen. None of our recipes depends on any of the potassium chloride salt replacements, although some of the special low-sodium ingredients use these in their processing. (Always check with your doctor before using a potassium chloride salt substitute.)

Every recipe provides the sodium content for the serving size. And to make it a little easier, we've organized the recipes in the chapter by sodium content—lowest at the start of the chapter to highest at the end of the chapter. You can choose all your favorites each day, knowing just how much sodium you're consuming. Or you can go online at idiotsguides.com/lowsodiumcooking to discover 2-week meal plans that allow you to eat within 1,000-milligram or 1,500-milligram limits simply and without fuss. Plus, you can follow the 2,000-milligram plan to step down your sodium intake gradually.

Equipped with essential information, you can cook and eat low sodium with confidence. Even if you need to restrict your sodium, you should never feel restricted in great taste and great company. With appetizing recipes, you can eat with your family and friends, communing over delicious dishes for everyday meals and special occasions alike.

Wishing you good health and good eating!

How This Book Is Organized

This book is divided into seven parts:

Part 1, In the Lo-So Know, provides the indispensable information on salt and sodium you need to know to eat and cook low-sodium meals. You learn how to read nutrition labels and find the sodium potentially hidden in your diet. We introduce you to salt alternatives and offer tips on how to add flavor to foods without using salt and other high-sodium seasonings and flavorings.

Part 2, Breakfasts and Brunches, offers foods for your early morning rush or your leisurely weekends.

Part 3, In the Lunchbox, provides recipes for your midday meal or any time you need a light bite. We give dozens of recipes for hearty salads, delicious dressings, filling soups and stews, and sodium-responsible sandwiches.

Part 4, Starters, Snacks, and Seasonings, features tempting recipes for appetizers, dips, snacks, and beverages. Also in this part we've included plenty of recipes to boost the flavor of your foods. Classic condiments, salsas, relishes, slathers, spreads, and seasoning blends help you add that bit of taste to make your meals memorable.

Part 5, Marvelous Main Dishes, highlights your needs for main dish recipes from simple to spectacular. You'll find everything from fish and seafood, chicken, turkey, beef, pork, and even vegetarian meals.

Part 6, Side by Side, is packed with recipes for all your favorite go-withs—breads, side salads, vegetables, and other side dishes that make your meals complete.

Finally, **Part 7, Sweet Treats and Sippers,** pleases your sweet tooth with recipes for scrumptious delights. Treat yourself to cookies, brownies, bars, fudges, sauces, puddings, cakes, cheesecakes, pies, tarts, crisps, cobblers, and indulgent beverages.

Garnishes

You'll see many sidebars throughout the book that offer you a little something extra. Here's what to look for:

DEFINITION

These sidebars offer definitions and provide helpful vocabulary for cooking low-sodium foods.

PINCH OF SAGE

These sidebars contain valuable information to help you in the kitchen and with specific recipes.

SALT PITFALL

These warnings tell you how to avoid eating or cooking with too much sodium.

But Wait! There's More!

Have you logged on to idiotsguides.com lately? If you haven't, go there now! As a bonus to the book, we've included additional resources, two-week menu plans, and more you'll want to check out, all online. Point your browser to idiotsguides.com/lowsodiumcooking, and enjoy!

Acknowledgments

Although only two names appear on the cover of this cookbook, we are all too aware of the contributions made by many others to make this book possible.

The authors would like to thank their families for their patience, for picking up some of the slack at home, for their child-care services, and for their willingness to taste-test everything.

We thank our fabulous agent Marilyn Allen of the Allen O'Shea Literary Agency for her support. Thank you, Mike Sanders, our original acquisitions editor who is now the associate publisher at Alpha. Thank you to our development editor Christy Wagner, who well deserved her promotion to senior development editor. And we thank both our original and current production editors Megan Douglass and Kayla Dugger and copy editors Nancy Wagner and Monica Stone for whipping our manuscripts into shape for accuracy and readability.

Trademarks

All terms mentioned in this book that are known to be or are suspected of being trademarks or service marks have been appropriately capitalized. Alpha Books and Penguin Group (USA) Inc. cannot attest to the accuracy of this information. Use of a term in this book should not be regarded as affecting the validity of any trademark or service mark.

In the Lo-So Know

With just a little helpful information, you can easily prepare sodium-sensible meals everyone will love—even those people not specifically watching their sodium intake. When you learn how to replace the salt shaker and other high-sodium seasonings and sauces with herbs and spices, veggies, fruits, and other seasoning secrets, you'll feel great about your reduced sodium levels and be savoring what you've cooked.

Additionally, you need to know which foods have naturally occurring sodium and in what amounts. More important, you should learn where sodium is hiding and which foods are available in a spectrum of reduced-sodium versions—and then where to find them. Once you've mastered this information—and it's easy, really it is—you'll have the confidence to step into your kitchen and create flavorful, mouthwatering meals to fit everyone's needs.

The Shakedown on Salt

In This Chapter

- Losing your taste for salt
- Is your water foiling your low-sodium efforts?
- Deciphering food labels
- Identifying sodium in disguise

Salty is one of the four basic tastes. Sodium, which salt can provide, is an essential mineral every body needs for regulating fluid balance. The amount of sodium the body requires, though, is very small—exceptionally less than the average person's intake.

If you're trying to cut back on salt and other sources of sodium, gathering some knowledge will help you obtain your goal. You need the basics: What is salt? Where does sodium come from? How can I cook without it? With answers to these questions, you can begin serving sodium-responsible meals that are not only healthful but also delicious and delectable.

What's Shakin'?

Common table salt, the chemical compound sodium chloride (NaCl), is a major source of the sodium most people consume. By weight, it's about 40 percent sodium and 60 percent chloride.

The average person doesn't need nearly the amount of sodium he or she eats. Do you know you can ingest all the sodium your body needs to maintain healthy functioning without eating a grain of salt? It's true. Sodium occurs naturally in the meats, dairy products, poultry, eggs, seafood, fruits, vegetables, and cereal products you consume; without even realizing it, you're taking in sodium, too.

Moreover, many processed foods are prepared with salt and sodium-rich ingredients. Diets built around convenience foods may be bloated with sodium that's harder to detect.

Salt at Work

The popularity of salt has endured throughout the ages because of its usefulness. Its preserving properties were vital before civilizations had readily accessible refrigeration. Adding salt to a food dehydrates the cells, including any bacteria cells present, which in turn retards bacterial growth that results in spoilage.

Salt is also the muscle behind the flour in bread making. The salt strengthens the gluten in the dough, thereby enabling the dough to expand with a uniform texture. You'll find that salt-free breads are coarser and denser in texture than typical fluffy white breads.

Salt provides a means for curing meats, pickling vegetables and other foods, and making cheese. But now, with today's technologies, manufacturers have developed alternative methods to making lunch meats, pickles, and cheeses without using salt. That means many of your favorite foods are available without skyrocketing sodium contents.

More important to you on a personal level, salt is the enduring flavor enhancer. In simple terms, your tongue tastes salt and sends a message to your brain. Your brain now knows you're eating, so it lets your nose in on the information. Your nose starts to smell the food. The flavor of the food comes from your tongue tasting and your nose smelling the food.

Retraining Your Taste Buds

You've probably spent any number of years honing your taste for salt. But the good news is that your taste for salt is developed and not innate! Because you've learned to like salty foods, you can *unlearn* your love of salt, too.

If you have the luxury, try cutting back on salt gradually. Take the salt shaker off the table, replace salt in recipes with herb-and-spice seasoning blends or other appropriate salt substitutes, and opt for the unsalted versions of snacks such as nuts and crackers. To help you step down your sodium intake, we've included a 2,000-milligram sodium per day meal plan online at idiotsguides.com/lowsodiumcooking. Over time, your taste for salt will diminish.

Keep the following tips in mind for reducing sodium in your diet until you reach a level comfortable for you that falls within your doctor's or nutritionist's guidelines, if necessary:

- Season foods without salt at the table and when cooking; try herbs, spices, and other low-sodium seasonings instead.

- Substitute low-sodium forms of seasonings and sauces, such as Worcestershire sauce, soy sauce, and bouillon.

- Purchase ingredients with the lowest sodium content possible by carefully reading the nutrition labels.

- Use fresh or frozen fruits and vegetables, or no-salt-added canned foods.

- Prepare pasta, noodles, rice, and hot cereals without the optional salt.

- Choose no-salt-added condiments, such as mustard, ketchup, barbecue sauce, and salsa.

PINCH OF SAGE

Now that you're not seasoning with salt, don't throw out the salt shaker! If you've spilled wine on a tablecloth, blot it up, then cover the stain with salt to absorb the remainder, and rinse the tablecloth with cold water. If the spill is on carpet, vacuum up the salt after it has absorbed the spill. To keep cut flowers fresh longer, add a dash of salt to the water. Sprinkle salt into canvas shoes to absorb moisture and odors. Rub tea- or coffee-stained cups with salt to remove the stains. Soak new candles in a strong salt solution for several hours and dry well to keep them from dripping when they burn.

It's Something in the Water

Sodium? In your water? It's true. Depending on the source, the sodium content of water varies greatly. If you're using tap water, the source of your water is your local water department. You can contact them for information on the sodium levels in your tap water. Well water users can have their water tested to determine the sodium content. Contact your local or state health department or well water professional.

One way to bypass your tap is to purchase a water filtration system. You can choose either a pitcher that filters out sodium, and keep it in your refrigerator for drinking and cooking needs, or you can install a filter on your kitchen tap that removes a percentage of the sodium from the tap water.

If you have a water softener in your home, the chemicals used to condition your water are likely raising its sodium content. Bypass your softener whenever you use water for drinking or cooking.

If your water's sodium content is too high for your needs, consider buying sodium-free bottled water for use in cooking and for drinking.

SALT PITFALL

We have based the recipes in this book on the use of sodium-free bottled water. Therefore, the nutrition analysis given for any recipe calling for water does not account for any water-supplied sodium.

Navigating the Nutrition Analysis

The nutrition analysis accompanying each recipe in this book can help you plan your daily meals and snacks to fall within your recommended sodium intake. You'll also be able to track your calories and sodium.

The amounts you'll find listed with each recipe refer to an individual serving, and with each recipe, we've provided the serving size. Should a recipe provide a range of servings along with a range in an ingredient amount, the information offered for each serving is based on the first serving size given in conjunction with the first ingredient amount listed.

If a recipe offers an alternative ingredient, it's not included in the nutrition analysis; we have used those ingredients listed first for the calculations. Likewise, the analyses do not take into account any suggested serving accompaniments, as you may or may not choose to use these suggestions.

We've included two nutrients in the analyses for each recipe: calories and sodium.

How many calories you need to consume each day depends on your gender, age, height, and physical activity level. Check with your doctor or nutritionist for the appropriate amount of calories you should eat. Per gram, protein and carbohydrate contain 4 calories while fat carries 9 calories. For additional information, visit choosemyplate.gov.

The current recommended sodium intake for healthy young adults from the 2010 Dietary Guidelines for Americans and the American Heart Association is 1,500 milligrams. This most recent release of Dietary Guidelines for Americans suggests lower intakes of 1,300 milligrams and 1,200 milligrams sodium are adequate for middle-age and elderly adults, respectively. The 2,300 milligrams sodium recommendation you may have been familiar with is now considered the Tolerable Upper Intake Level (UL) for sodium intake. If your doctor or nutritionist has indicated a modified amount for you, follow those instructions.

Please use these nutrition analyses as guidelines. Differences in your exact ingredients and preparation methods may result in altered nutrient amounts. A food's nutritional values can vary by season, grower, and location. Thereby, the provided figures cannot be exact. Still, you can trust that the numbers are close and use them for tracking your intake.

What's more, you may need to substitute various ingredients to follow the recommendations provided by your doctor or nutritionist. Or you may be unable to find a particular ingredient, such as salt-free whole-wheat bread, and need to substitute the available salt-free white bread. Likewise, you may enjoy experimenting with ingredient substitutions for herbs and spices, vinegars, oils, or vegetables. These adaptations may tweak a recipe to fall within your family's eating habits, provide needed variety, or use available ingredients without significantly altering the nutritional value of the recipe.

Reading Food Labels

Nutrition labels contain the information you need to know about the foods you buy. The best place to start sleuthing through nutrition labels is in your own pantry and refrigerator. You'll usually find the nutrition facts for a product on the back or side of a food package. At the top or beginning of the box, you'll find the serving size for that food. If you scroll down or over a little, you'll see sodium listed. The number of sodium milligrams in each serving follows. To the far right is a percentage. The percentage of sodium given is based on a 2,000-calorie diet for a healthy adult. (This number may not be of value to you.)

Going through the foods already in your home can prove to be eye-opening. You may discover foods high in sodium that you never would have suspected. You'll certainly discover some staples you need to replace with low-sodium alternatives.

When searching for low-sodium products, you'll need to compare nutrition labels. Unfortunately, you can't just glance at the number of sodium milligrams. When you evaluate similar foods, first note the serving sizes. If they're the same, you can simply compare the amount of sodium in each. If the serving sizes differ, you'll have to do some math. A product with a serving size of 1 cup containing 100 milligrams sodium is actually lower in sodium than a similar product with a serving size of 6 ounces containing 80 milligrams sodium.

> **SALT PITFALL**
>
> When you're looking for low-sodium food, beware of the following salty terms that might appear on food labels or restaurant menus: *pickled, brined, cured, smoked, corned, seasoned, breaded, au gratin, barbecued,* and *canned.*

Finding appropriate foods to eat that allow you to comply with your low-sodium needs takes time and patience. The good news is that after a short time, you will find suitable replacements for the foods you normally eat. Then, you'll only have to play sleuth again when you require a new ingredient.

Understanding FDA Guidelines

The U.S. Food and Drug Administration (FDA) has guidelines in place for food manufacturers that can help you more easily identify sodium-sensible foods. Labels can carry specific terms based on their sodium content. Unfortunately, it isn't always cut and dried. Some products use *low-sodium* generically, even though they may be "very low-sodium" according to the guidelines. Labels that read *reduced sodium* may be reduced by more than 25 percent; these labels typically indicate the higher percentage.

Use the sodium-related label terms listed in the following table to locate the products on store shelves or in online catalogs. Then, read those labels for exact information.

FDA Sodium Guidelines

Term	What It Means
Sodium free	Less than 5 milligrams sodium per serving
Very low sodium	35 milligrams or less sodium per serving
Low sodium	140 milligrams or less sodium per serving
Light in sodium	Usual sodium level is reduced by at least 50 percent
Reduced sodium	Usual sodium level is reduced by 25 percent
Unsalted, no-salt-added, or *without added salt*	Made without the salt that's normally used, but still contains the sodium that's a natural part of the food itself

Salt by Any Other Name

When you're in the thick of reading an ingredients list, you need to keep an eye out for all forms of sodium. These may be listed as sodium, sodium alginate, sodium sulfite, sodium caseinate, disodium phosphate, sodium benzoate, sodium hydroxide, monosodium glutamate (*MSG*), sodium citrate, baking powder, baking soda, sodium bicarbonate, Na, and more.

> **DEFINITION**
>
> **MSG,** or monosodium glutamate, occurs naturally in many foods, but the manufactured version is used as an added flavor enhancer. MSG contains about a third the amount of sodium found in table salt. You should be particularly vigilant when eating Chinese foods, which frequently contain MSG as a flavor enhancer.

Reality check! You're not going to memorize every sodium-containing compound that may be listed on a food label. So just keep it simple. Look for the word *sodium*. It may be listed individually or within another word. Other ingredients you need to watch for are *salt*, *baking powder*, and *baking soda*. MSG is also troublesome, as the abbreviation keeps you from spotting the sodium portion of the ingredient, but that's what that *S* stands for.

Regardless of how any sodium-rich ingredient is listed, you can always refer to the nutrition facts. Every milligram of sodium will be accounted for in that amount.

The Least You Need to Know

- Sodium is an essential mineral, but you can easily meet your body's needs without using the salt shaker.
- The taste for salt is learned, so you can teach your taste buds to enjoy less salty foods.
- Choose sodium-free bottled water for drinking and cooking if your tap water is too high in sodium.
- Food labels offer clues to sodium content, but you have to read the nutrition label to get the hard facts.

Kitchen Salternatives

In This Chapter

- Deciphering commercially prepared salt substitutes
- Flavoring with herbs and spices
- Seasoning with fruits, vegetables, and liquid flavorings
- Choosing the right butter or margarine for you
- Baking with sodium-free leavening agents

Your doctor or nutritionist advised you to stop adding salt to your foods during and after cooking. Now, you're standing in your kitchen empty-handed and at a loss. How do you cook without salt? Fortunately, the answer is *deliciously!* You can still create flavorful meals without adding salt. You just need a little know-how.

If your doctor or nutritionist has indicated that any of the commercially prepared salt substitutes are appropriate for you, all you have to do is pick up some at the supermarket. In addition, you can employ the great flavors of herbs, spices, fruits, vegetables, oils, vinegars, syrups, and sweeteners.

If you think cooking without salt will result in bland, tasteless foods, hold on to your fork! Once you learn how to introduce flavor without the aid of your salt shaker, you'll be amazed how you can whip up delectable, sumptuous foods your family and friends will devour without saying, "Pass the salt, please!"

Close Encounters of the Three Kindas

While perusing the spice aisle at your local supermarket, you'll find—there, just below eye level—three different alternatives to salt: lite salt, salt substitute, and herb and spice blends. (Check with your doctor or nutritionist to learn which ones are suitable for you.)

Worth Half Its Salt

As the name implies, *lite salt* does contain salt. You can use the half-and-half mixture of salt (sodium chloride) and potassium chloride in cooking and baking as well as for seasoning at the table.

Lite salt may contain potassium iodide, as do some regular salts. Salt is often iodized for dietary purposes. Iodine deficiency can cause a condition of the thyroid gland called goiter.

Potassium Imposters

Salt substitute is the term applied to the potassium chloride product used to replace ordinary salt. A salt substitute contains no sodium. You can use it in cooking and for seasoning at the table.

> **DEFINITION**
>
> **Lite salt** is a blend of sodium chloride and potassium chloride in equal parts. Because salt makes up only half the mixture, lite salt contains 50 percent less sodium than regular salt. **Salt substitute** is a product intended for people on sodium-restricted diets; comprised of potassium chloride, salt substitutes are sodium free. Check with your doctor before using any salt replacement containing potassium chloride or salt substitute.

Some people dislike potassium chloride salt alternatives because of their bitter aftertaste. Some salt substitutes claim to have no bitter aftertaste. Taste-test them yourself to see which ones you like.

Herb and Spice Blends

Also available for those trying to reduce their sodium intake are herb and spice blends. These salt-free salt substitute seasoning blends are available in a wide range of flavors to season any number of dishes. You can use them in place of salt in recipes as well as for at-the-table seasoning.

Because herbs and spices contain trace amounts of sodium, these seasoning blends aren't entirely sodium free. However, the slight amount of sodium in the portions used shouldn't cause concern.

Many foods naturally contain sodium. As a matter of fact, your body requires sodium to function properly. Your doctor or nutritionist can recommend the proper sodium intake for you.

Flavor Savers

Preparing flavorful, mouthwatering foods without added salt—and even without a potassium chloride salt substitute—is possible. You can infuse flavor into recipes through a plethora of ingredients. Herbs, spices, fruits, vegetables, oils, vinegars, syrups, and sweeteners can all perk up the taste of food.

Herb Insight

Use herbs in cooking in either their fresh or dried forms. Many people prefer the bright flavor of fresh herbs to their dried counterparts. Fresh herbs need gentle treatment, though. You may store them in the refrigerator for up to 5 days. If you need to hold fresh herbs longer, place them stem end down in a tall glass of cold water in the refrigerator, and change the water every other day.

High-moisture fresh herbs such as basil, mint, tarragon, and chives can be frozen to preserve their fresh taste—although freezing makes them limp when they thaw. Wash and pat dry the herbs before spreading individual leaves on a baking sheet. Place the sheet in the freezer until the leaves are frozen solid. Transfer them to a zipper-lock freezer bag, and store in the freezer. When needed, use the same amount of frozen herbs as you would fresh herbs.

Dried herbs offer the convenience of a long shelf life—most can be stored for up to 6 months. For a quick test of your herb's freshness, open the jar. If you can't identify the herb by its smell, replace it. Store your herbs in a cool, dark place because sunlight and heat cause dried herbs to deteriorate more quickly. Don't store your herb jars next to the stove.

Herbs offer a wide variety of aromas and flavors. Experiment to discover your own favorite food-herb pairings. Here are some traditional uses for common herbs:

Basil enhances the taste of tomato dishes and sauces, as well as soups, salads, pastas, and meats. It's frequently used in Italian and other Mediterranean cuisines.

Bay leaves infuse flavor into soups, stews, and marinades. Discard these large, brittle leaves before serving.

Cilantro, the leaf of the coriander plant, is a traditional ingredient in Mexican and Indian dishes, as well as in Caribbean and Asian cooking. Try it in salsas, sauces, soups, stews, salads, and meats. It's sometimes referred to as Chinese parsley because it resembles flat-leaf parsley.

Dill weed's feathery green leaves liven up vegetables, salads, eggs, light meats, fish, mustards, and other sauces. It's used extensively in Scandinavian cooking.

Marjoram is sweeter than oregano and widely used in French, Italian, North African, and Middle Eastern cuisines. It seasons meats, poultry, fish, beans, breads, cheese dishes, eggs, tomato dishes, soups, and salad dressings.

PINCH OF SAGE

Dried herbs pack a more concentrated flavor than fresh herbs, so you'll have to adjust the amount used. A good rule is 1 tablespoon fresh herb equals 1 teaspoon dried herb. You can adjust the amounts to taste, of course.

Mint is available in a variety of types, with peppermint and spearmint being the most common. Use mint in beverages, candies, baked goods, desserts, vegetables, salads, jellies, and lamb sauce.

Oregano is more savory than marjoram and used regularly in Italian cooking. Use oregano to enhance pizzas, sauces, salads, eggs, meats, and vegetables.

Parsley is available in curly and flat-leaf varieties, with the latter being more flavorful. Parsley is mild enough to be added to nearly any recipe. It's often used for color.

Rosemary's gray-green, piney leaves complement Italian, Greek, and Provençal recipes. Use it in breads, eggs, meats, potatoes and other vegetables, soups, and stews. It's often called for in its ground form.

Sage is a strong-flavored herb, so use its green-gray leaves or dried form in moderation. Breads, dressings, sausages, and pork all benefit from its distinctive taste.

Tarragon is prized in French cuisine. Use it in sauces, salads, and fish and poultry dishes.

Thyme is called for in herbes de Provence, bouquet garni, zahtar (a Middle Eastern spice blend), jerk seasonings, and curry blends. Try it in pizzas, potatoes and other veggies, salads, soups, stews, eggs, meats, and dressings.

Spice It Up

Spices can kick up the flavor of any number of dishes. If you opt for spices in their ground forms, store them in a cool, dry place. If heat and moisture are kept at bay, ground spices will stay fresh for about 6 months. If you prefer to grind your own whole spices, you can store the whole spices for a year or longer, as you can dry mustard. If you have slightly older spices and you just can't be wasteful, add a bit more than the recipes call for.

Spice blends are readily available for purchase. Some of your favorites may contain salt as an ingredient, though. Whether you choose to mix your own spice blends because you need to avoid the salt or because it's more economical, store them as you would any other spice or herb. Glass jars with tight-fitting lids are your best option. Keep them in the same cool, dry, dark place you store the remainder of your collection.

The heady aromas and sharp tastes of spices can invigorate your cooking. Use the following common spices to expand the flavor of your foods. But don't feel you have to work within these perimeters. Feel free to experiment with your favorite flavors.

Allspice has an aroma that hints of cloves, nutmeg, and cinnamon—hence the name. Use it in baked goods, beverages, meats, poultry, grains, egg dishes, soups, and stews.

Anise seeds taste and smell like licorice. They flavor baked goods, candies, breads, cheeses, fish and shellfish, sausages, and condiments.

Caraway seeds give rye bread its distinctive flavor. You can use them to season cabbage, potatoes, soups, stews, sausages, and cheeses.

Cayenne is sometimes labeled as ground red pepper. Its hot zing can add flavor to beans, meats, chilis, soups, stews, sauces, and dips.

Celery seeds are tiny brown seeds with a celery-like flavor and aroma. Use them in moderation on eggs, poultry, dressings, salads, salad dressings, tomato dishes, stews, and sauces.

Chili powder is a spice blend of ground chiles, paprika, cumin, and garlic. Many blends include salt as an ingredient, so watch out for those. As its name implies, it's most often used in chilis, but you may also add it to dips, sauces, corn breads, beans, meats, and chicken.

 SALT PITFALL

When purchasing any spice blends such as chili powder, curry powder, and poultry seasoning, read the labels and ingredient lists carefully. Many use salt or even MSG as an ingredient. If the labels aren't clear, you may have to contact the manufacturer for details.

Chinese five-spice powder is a mixture of star anise, fennel or anise seeds, Szechwan or black peppercorns, cinnamon, and cloves or ginger. Use it to season Asian dishes, meats, poultry, and stir-fries.

Cinnamon is used in traditional Mexican cooking. You'll also find it useful for baked goods, beverages, sweet potatoes, pumpkin and squash dishes, sauces, and curries.

Cloves in their whole form resemble small spikes and while they'll add flavor to dishes when used whole, be sure to discard the spiky bits before serving. Use whole or ground cloves to enhance baked goods, fruits, sweet vegetables, pork, sauces, and ketchup.

Coriander seeds' sweet-tart citrus taste can spice up meats, eggs, dips, sauces, marinades, grains, and cream soups.

Cumin, prized in Indian, Thai, Vietnamese, and Mexican cuisines, can be used in seed or ground form. Try it in beans, chilis, and curries.

Curry powder is a spice blend that may consist of cumin, turmeric, coriander, fennel, cinnamon, cloves, and so on. The flavors range from mild to fiery hot. You can add a blend to chicken or tuna salad, soups, eggs, and vegetables.

Dry mustard allows you to make your own low-sodium mustards. It's also good for eggs, cheese dishes, meats, and salad dressings.

Ginger can be added to Asian dishes in its fresh form. Ground ginger is commonly used in baked goods, beverages, and curries.

Nutmeg and its more intense lacy outer covering, *mace*, are typically added to baked goods. Nutmeg lends flavor to sauces, beverages, custards, and puddings as well. You can also try it for savory dishes of meat, chicken, fish, vegetables, soups, and stews.

Paprika is ground from the pimiento, the pepper used to stuff green olives. Most commercial paprika is mild, but hot versions do exist. What you find on your supermarket shelf and what's called for in most recipes is the mild version, unless otherwise noted. Use it to liven up goulashes, chicken, fish, eggs, potatoes, soups, and stews.

Pepper is available in white, green, and black peppercorns, whole or ground. It's a staple spice around the world, and you can use it in nearly every savory dish.

Poppy seeds are tiny, round, blue-gray seeds from the opium poppy flower. Sprinkle them on breads, rolls, and noodles or into salad dressings and dips.

Poultry seasoning is a blend of spices and herbs such as sage, thyme, rosemary, marjoram, parsley, black pepper, onion powder, garlic powder, and nutmeg. Watch for blends that contain salt. Its use is evident from its name.

Sesame seeds are valued in Asian and Middle Eastern cuisines. Embed these seeds atop breads, rolls, and crackers, or scatter them in salads or stir-fries.

Turmeric is a golden-yellow spice that easily stains. Try it in rice, chutneys, relishes, and curry powders.

Good Ol' Fruits and Veggies

What could be more basic than flavoring foods with other foods? At times, it's difficult to distinguish whether an ingredient is a main ingredient or a flavoring, but don't fuss too much over it. As long as the eatin' is good, go with it. However, if you're looking for a new depth of flavor for a recipe, try adding a seasoning fruit or vegetable such as the following:

Bell peppers are available in a rainbow of colors. Green bell peppers are immature and have a more raw taste. Red, orange, and yellow bell peppers are milder and sweeter. Use minced, diced, and chopped bell peppers in egg dishes, meats, chicken, fish, beans, cheese dishes, tomato dishes, potatoes and other vegetables, soups, stews, chilis, grains, pastas, salads, sauces, and dips.

Celery is commonly added to dishes for flavor, but it's fairly high in sodium, as vegetables go. One large rib of celery has about 50 milligrams sodium, so add it in moderation. Sliced, diced, and chopped celery enhances the taste of egg dishes, cheese dishes, fish, beans, soups, stews, tomato dishes, potatoes and other vegetables, grains, pastas, dressings, salads, sauces, dips, and more.

Chili peppers pack a heat that can kick up the flavor for fiery food lovers. The capsaicin that accounts for the heat of a chili pepper is concentrated in the white ribs as well as the seeds, so removing these veins and seeds from the inside of the pepper reduces the burn factor.

SALT PITFALL

Very important: thoroughly wash your hands after handling hot peppers or consider wearing gloves. You won't want to rub your eye with the essence of the pepper still on your fingers!

Garlic is a pungent but delicious addition to many dishes. Buy fresh garlic bulbs or prepared garlic cloves, chopped garlic, minced garlic, or crushed garlic. The flavor of fresh garlic is stronger, but prepared garlic is very convenient. You can use garlic powder in cooking, but don't substitute it for fresh garlic.

Lemon juice and zest add a bright, citrusy zing to recipes. Fresh lemon juice and zest are superior in flavor, but you can substitute bottled lemon juice and grated lemon peel from the spice aisle if convenience is a priority. Of course, other citrus juices and zests are just as valuable, including lime, orange, and grapefruit.

Mushrooms come in large variety and a wide price range. Button mushrooms, with their small white caps, are common in supermarkets. Portobello mushrooms, including baby portobellos (also known as crimini mushrooms), are also largely available. You may also find shiitake, oyster, morel, and other mushrooms offered in their fresh or dried forms. (Unless you're an expert, do not gather wild mushrooms for cooking.)

Onions introduce an array of flavors from pungent to sweet, mild to sharp. Scallions, green onions, shallots, red onions, yellow onions, white onions, sweet onions—your choices are plentiful. You can enhance almost any savory recipe, from breads to soups, salads to sauces, and meats to grains, with the addition of onions.

PINCH OF SAGE

The age-old question: how do you keep your eyes dry when cutting an onion? Try chilling your peeled onion for a bit before chopping it. You should also cut into the root end last.

Raisins come in two basic varieties: golden and dark. You're probably most familiar with the dark raisins your mom gave you as a snack. Both are made from Thompson seedless grapes, so use whichever type you prefer. Raisins can sweeten up breads, baked goods, desserts, grains, salads, and meats.

Tomatoes, in either their fresh or dried forms, lend their flavor to an array of recipes. Try them in egg dishes, meats, poultry, fish, dips, beans, vegetables, soups, stews, chilis, chowders, breads, grains, pastas, salads, and sauces.

Making a Splash

Liquid flavorings give you another option for great taste in place of salt. Try these:

Honey is often thought of as a replacement for sugar, but the colors and flavors of honey range based on which flowers the bees visited. Generally, light-colored honey is milder, and darker honeys have a bolder taste. Honey can add flavor to sauces, salad dressings, marinades, beverages, breads, desserts, and baked goods.

SALT PITFALL

Do not give honey to children younger than 12 months of age because botulism spores can be present in honey. Infants' digestive systems may be too immature to digest the bacterial spores, which can make the babies sick.

Maple syrup comes in light, medium, and dark ambers, with the tastes ranging from delicate to mapley to robust. Keep a good-quality maple syrup in your refrigerator to enhance meats, chicken, beans, vegetables, baked goods, and desserts.

Molasses adds a distinct taste to meats, poultry, fish, vegetables, sauces, and baked goods.

Oil comes in a wide variety of types. Olive, peanut, sesame, walnut, and avocado oils provide great tastes. Salad dressings will have subtle flavor changes if you substitute another oil. Stir-fries and vegetables may also benefit from oil experimentation.

Vanilla extract, along with the various other extracts found in your spice aisle, quickly flavors baked goods, sauces, vegetables, and beverages.

Vinegar comes in several varieties, including white, cider, red wine, balsamic, rice, and numerous other flavored vinegars. Splash it in marinades, salad dressings, potato salads, egg dishes, seafood, cabbage, leafy greens, tomato sauces, mustards, and pastas. When opting for rice vinegar, be careful which bottle you grab. Choose the sodium-free version because the regular type is loaded with sodium.

The Better Butter

We've used always-sodium-free unsalted butter in preparing the recipes in this book. It's widely available; look for it in your grocer's dairy case, labeled "unsalted." Salted and unsalted butters are interchangeable in most recipes. You'll want to purchase the unsalted type for your dietary needs.

If you're watching your saturated fat and cholesterol intake, choose a sodium-sensible margarine. Talk to your doctor or nutritionist about sodium content, saturated fat, cholesterol amounts, trans-fatty acids, and other concerns that may affect your butter or margarine choice. He or she can recommend the right butter or margarine for you.

SALT PITFALL

Baked goods should be prepared with a margarine that contains at least 60 percent fat. Spreads lower in fat cannot be used for baking purposes.

If you do substitute for the unsalted butter, calculate the additional sodium, decreased fats, and change in calories. You can compare nutrition labels at the supermarket or go to nutritiondata.self.com for nutrition facts.

Leavening Agent Awareness

Two of the most common leavening agents used in baked goods are baking powder and baking soda. They work great in giving your baked goods the rise they need. The bad news: both are high-sodium products. The good news: sodium-free substitutions are available. If you can't find them locally, order them from a reputable online store.

One option is Hain Pure Foods' Featherweight Baking Powder. This sodium-free baking powder is a blend of monocalcium phosphate, potato starch, and potassium bicarbonate. Add this product to a recipe just as you would regular baking powder.

If your doctor or nutritionist indicates you shouldn't have the 70 milligrams potassium in the $\frac{1}{8}$-teaspoon serving of the Featherweight Baking Powder, try Ener-G Baking Powder. This sodium-free product is a blend of calcium carbonate and citric acid. A note of warning: the Ener-G Baking Powder is a single-acting product, unlike the standard double-acting regular baking powder you may be used to. You'll need to use nearly twice the amount of the single-acting baking powder as the regular baking powder called for in the recipe. Additionally, you may have to tweak the recipe to add the baking powder at the end of mixing and get your pan into the oven quickly. Read the label carefully for specific instructions.

Ener-G also sells a sodium-free baking soda that's simply calcium carbonate and magnesium carbonate. Its label advises using twice the amount of regular baking soda called for in a recipe.

You may come across recipes that call for cream of tartar. Frontier makes a cream of tartar product that has just 1 milligram sodium in a ½-teaspoon serving. It's marketed as an activator for the Hain Featherweight Baking Powder.

SALT PITFALL

Recipes in this book that call for sodium-free baking powder or sodium-free baking soda call for the equivalent of the original measurement of regular baking powder and baking soda. If you're using Featherweight Baking Powder, simply add the amount indicated in the recipe. If you choose Ener-G Baking Powder, nearly double the measurement. When using Ener-G Baking Soda, double the measurement. Carefully read the label directions for any other sodium-free substitutions you may use.

The Least You Need to Know

- Seasoning without salt can create delicious dishes.
- Herbs and spices infuse flavor to make mouthwatering recipes, and you can kick up the taste of foods by seasoning with other foods, such as onions, garlic, and lemon juice.
- Low-sodium liquid flavorings, such as vinegars and concentrated extracts, are smart options for great taste.
- Unsalted butter reduces the sodium count in dishes, but ask your doctor or nutritionist about a sodium-sensible margarine substitute right for you.
- Read the label of a sodium-free leavening agent carefully for special directions on how to use that particular product.

Breakfasts and Brunches

Breakfast is the most important meal of the day and can help you start your day right with high energy and good nutrients. Taking the time to eat breakfast or brunch can boost your metabolism and help maintain your good health—all without tallying up too much sodium.

Whether it's a rushed weekday morning or a leisurely weekend morning, taking the time to make and eat breakfast, or lounge around the kitchen table and enjoy a homemade brunch with your family, your day will be better off for it.

Fast-Fix Breakfasts

In This Chapter

- Starting your day right
- Planning for the most important meal of the day
- Being sodium wise in a time crunch
- Preparing quick, low-sodium breakfasts

From the moment your morning wake-up alarm sounds to the time you arrive at work or school, you're playing a game of beat the clock. You may think you've tricked time, shaving off minutes by skipping breakfast, but the trick's on you.

Without a nutritious start to your day, your energy level languishes, your attention span shrivels, your blood sugar level crashes, and your metabolism rebels. The best way to avoid these downfalls is to find a way to squeeze good nutrition into your morning rush.

The recipes in this chapter offer you some possibilities for doing just that. You may need a fast-fix, quick-eat breakfast. Or maybe you're really pressed for time and need a speedy breakfast that can travel with you. Either way, we're here to make you a believer in breakfast!

Making a Breakfast Plan

You plan for the future; you plan for a rainy day; you even plan what to have for dinner. But when it comes to the meal that jump-starts your day, do you have a strategy? You don't need a spreadsheet or a computer-generated, color-coded bar chart. You just need a simple grocery list. Because if you have the necessary ingredients on hand, you can whip up a sodium-sensible breakfast faster than you can say "hitting the drive-thru."

If your idea of fitting breakfast into the whirlwind you call morning is grabbing a prepared pastry or greasy breakfast sandwich through your car window, you're going to have to rethink your routine. And forget about the astronomical sodium content those tastiest of morning temptations contain because they're all-around lacking in nutrition. You and your body deserve better. Plus, in the time you spend repeating your order into a crackling speaker, you can prepare a homemade, sodium-mindful meal.

If you just don't feel like cooking first thing in the morning, you have a few ready-made backup options. Choose shredded wheat, puffed wheat, or puffed rice cereal over other regular ready-to-eat cereals. Avoid instant hot cereals that soar in sodium. Instead, choose quick oats, creamy hot wheat cereals, or farina (ground wheat berries). With these in hand, you have all the time and options you need for a fast, healthful breakfast.

PINCH OF SAGE

If you don't care for the mainstream, ready-to-eat cereals that fit your sodium-restricted diet, check your supermarket's cereal aisle for a few low-sodium and very low-sodium alternatives. (These cereals tend to have healthy-sounding brands and names.)

Peanut Butter Stacked Apple

A crunchy apple spread with creamy peanut butter gives you a quick morning kick-start.

Yield:	Prep time:	Serving size:
1 serving	3 minutes	1 apple

Each serving has:		
325.1 calories	0 mg sodium	

1 large apple

2 TB. no-salt-added natural peanut butter

1. Core apple, and slice horizontally into 4 or 5 sections.
2. Spread peanut butter between apple sections, and reassemble apple.

PINCH OF SAGE

Good apple varieties to try in this recipe are Gala, McIntosh, Red Delicious, and Empire.

Peanut Butter and Pineapple Burrito

Smooth peanut butter and sweet pineapple are wrapped up in a tender tortilla.

Yield:	Prep time:	Serving size:
1 serving	3 minutes	1 burrito
Each serving has:		
483.7 calories	2.9 mg sodium	

2 TB. no-salt-added natural peanut butter

2 TB. crushed pineapple

1 Fresh Tortilla (recipe in Chapter 19) or other low-sodium tortilla

1. In a small bowl, stir together peanut butter and pineapple.

2. Spread mixture down center of Fresh Tortilla. Fold up tortilla burrito-style.

PINCH OF SAGE

Oil separation is normal in natural peanut butter, so don't pour it off! Instead, stir the oil back into the peanut butter. You also need to refrigerate natural peanut butter after opening it to prevent rancidity because it doesn't contain preservatives. Tightly closed, you can store it for up to 3 months.

Peach Melba Oatmeal

Juicy peaches and raspberries sweeten every bite of this smooth morning oatmeal.

Yield:	Prep time:	Cook time:	Serving size:
1½ cups	4 minutes	1½ minutes	¾ cup
Each serving has:			
201 calories	3.6 mg sodium		

½ cup quick oats

1 cup water

⅓ cup chopped frozen peach slices

¼ cup frozen raspberries

1 TB. granulated sugar

1 tsp. fat-free milk

1. Pour oats into a medium microwave-safe bowl, and add water. Add peaches and raspberries, and microwave on high for $1\frac{1}{2}$ to 2 minutes or until oats are softened and liquid is absorbed. Stir to combine.

2. Stir in sugar and milk, and mix well.

Salternative: If you prefer to use fresh fruit, you can still follow this recipe as is, or for a crisper texture, stir the fresh peaches and raspberries into the oatmeal after it's cooked.

Spiced Apple-Cranberry Steel-Cut Oats

Slow-cooked, slightly chewy steel-cut oats mingle with tender apples and cranberries in this sweet and spicy mixture.

Yield:	Prep time:	Cook time:	Serving size:
5 cups	5 minutes	8 hours	1 cup
Each serving has:			
214.4 calories	5.2 mg sodium		

2 cups peeled, cored, and finely chopped Gala apples (about 3 medium)

$\frac{1}{2}$ cup halved cranberries, fresh or frozen

1 TB. fresh lemon juice

1 cup steel-cut oats

2 tsp. ground cinnamon

$\frac{1}{2}$ tsp. ground nutmeg

$\frac{1}{4}$ tsp. ground cloves

$2\frac{1}{2}$ cups water

2 cups natural apple juice

1. Coat a $3\frac{1}{2}$- to 5-quart slow cooker with nonstick cooking spray.

2. In a medium bowl, combine apples, cranberries, and lemon juice, stirring to coat evenly.

3. In a large bowl, stir together steel-cut oats, apple mixture, cinnamon, nutmeg, cloves, water, and apple juice. Transfer to the prepared slow cooker.

4. Cover and cook on low for 8 hours or until oats are tender. Stir to blend before serving.

PINCH OF SAGE

Fresh cranberries are available only in late fall. Place an extra bag in your freezer to have cranberries on hand throughout the remainder of the year.

Honey Nut Multi-Grain Cereal

Enjoy a creamy whole-grain cereal sweetened with honey and with the added mild crunch of pecans.

Yield:	Prep time:	Cook time:	Serving size:
1 serving	3 minutes	1½ minutes	1 bowl

Each serving has:		
305 calories	11.4 mg sodium	

¾ cup water

½ cup sodium-free multi-grain hot cereal (rye, barley, oats, and wheat)

1 TB. honey

1 TB. fat-free milk

2 TB. chopped unsalted pecans

1. In a small microwave-safe bowl, pour water over cereal. Microwave on high for 1½ to 2 minutes or until done.

2. Stir in honey, milk, and pecans until blended.

Salternative: Save a little sodium by replacing the milk with nondairy creamer if you like. You can substitute your favorite unsalted nuts for the pecans; try walnuts, peanuts, or even hazelnuts.

PINCH OF SAGE

If you're unsure whether a container is suitable for microwave use, test it first. Place 1 cup tap water and the container in your microwave oven, and microwave on high for 1 minute. The water should get warm and the container should be cool or lukewarm. If it's hot, it's not microwave-safe.

ILLINOIS PRAIRIE DISTRICT LIBRARY

Very Berry Tofu Breakfast Smoothie

Mixed sweet berries are delivered in a cool, frothy drink.

Yield:	Prep time:	Serving size:
2 cups	5 minutes	1 smoothie
Each serving has:		
341.6 calories	16.9 mg sodium	

6 oz. soft tofu, drained and chopped	¼ tsp. vanilla extract
6 ice cubes	¼ cup blueberries
3 TB. honey	¼ cup blackberries
	4 medium strawberries, hulled

1. In a blender, combine tofu, ice cubes, honey, vanilla extract, blueberries, blackberries, and strawberries.

2. Blend on high speed for 1 minute or until smooth, stopping to scrape down sides as necessary.

PINCH OF SAGE

This healthful drink starts your morning off right with lots of protein, calcium, and antioxidants—all in one convenient to-go cup.

Maple Syrup and Brown Sugar Oatmeal

Start your day with smooth oatmeal sweetened with a hint of maple goodness.

Yield:	Prep time:	Cook time:	Serving size:
1 serving	3 minutes	1 minute	1 bowl
Each serving has:			
413 calories	18.5 mg sodium		

½ cup quick oats	1 TB. pure maple syrup
¾ cup water	1 TB. fat-free milk
1 TB. firmly packed light brown sugar	

1. Pour oats into a small microwave-safe bowl. Add water, and microwave on high for 1 to 1½ minutes or until oats are softened and liquid is absorbed. Stir.

2. Stir in light brown sugar and maple syrup.

3. Stir in milk until well mixed.

Salternative: This recipe makes a thick oatmeal. If you prefer a thinner oatmeal, add ¼ to ½ cup more water, increasing the cooking time as necessary.

SALT PITFALL

Commercial instant oatmeals boast convenience, but they're loaded with sodium. Quick oats are a smart alternative—all as fast as instant with just a fraction of the sodium. Plus, you can create your own favorite flavors.

Wild Rice and Berries

Enjoy the *al dente* taste of wild rice topped with fresh blueberries.

Yield:	Prep time:	Serving size:
1 serving	3 minutes	1 bowl
Each serving has:		
136 calories	36.6 mg sodium	

½ cup cooked wild rice, chilled   Pinch ground cinnamon
¼ cup fresh blueberries   ¼ cup fat-free milk
½ tsp. honey

1. In a cereal bowl, combine wild rice, blueberries, honey, cinnamon, and milk.

2. Stir to mix well.

Salternative: You may serve this as a warm cereal, if you prefer. Warm the mixture in a small saucepan over low heat or in the microwave on reheat for 1 or 2 minutes or until heated through.

PINCH OF SAGE

With leftover wild rice, breakfast is as easy as stirring. Be sure to cook extra wild rice whenever you prepare it and store it in the refrigerator for a quick breakfast the next morning.

Creamy Morning Mixed Berries

Honey-kissed yogurt dresses fresh, juicy berries topped with a crunch.

Yield:	Prep time:	Serving size:
1 cup	5 minutes	1 cup
Each serving has:		
169.1 calories	38.5 mg sodium	

¼ cup plain fat-free yogurt	⅓ cup fresh blackberries
1 tsp. honey	1 TB. chopped unsalted walnuts
⅓ cup fresh blueberries	1 TB. ground flaxseed
⅓ cup fresh raspberries	

1. In a medium bowl, stir together yogurt and honey until blended.

2. Stir in blueberries, raspberries, and blackberries until evenly coated.

3. Sprinkle walnuts and flaxseed over top to serve.

PINCH OF SAGE

Ground flaxseed and walnuts are both good sources of the omega-3 fatty acid alpha linolenic acid (ALA). Store both in the refrigerator for freshness, or in the freezer for up to 6 months for an even longer shelf-life.

Overnight Maple and Brown Sugar Steel-Cut Oats

Chewy steel-cut oats are served up creamy with a sweet maple addition.

Yield:	Prep time:	Cook time:	Serving size:
1 serving	10 minutes, plus overnight cooling	10 minutes	1 bowl

Each serving has:			
270 calories	68.2 mg sodium		

¼ cup steel-cut oats

½ cup fat-free milk

½ cup water

1 TB. pure maple syrup

1 tsp. firmly packed dark brown sugar

1. In a small nonstick saucepan with a lid, combine steel-cut oats, milk, and water. Heat, uncovered, over high heat for 3 minutes or until milk begins boiling, stirring constantly to scrape the bottom of the saucepan to prevent scorching and boiling over.

2. Reduce heat to low. Simmer for 2 minutes, stirring slowly to scrape the bottom of the saucepan to prevent scorching.

3. Remove from heat. Stir often to prevent milk from sticking to the bottom of the saucepan and to cool, about 8 minutes. Cover with the lid and refrigerate overnight.

4. Uncover and heat over high heat for 3 minutes or until milk boils, slowly stirring constantly and scraping the bottom of the saucepan to prevent scorching.

5. Turn off heat, stir in maple syrup and dark brown sugar, and serve hot.

Salternative: Omit the maple syrup and/or dark brown sugar, and stir in fresh fruits and berries, honey, ground cinnamon, chopped unsalted nuts, ground flaxseeds, a pat of butter, or your favorite oatmeal toppings.

PINCH OF SAGE

To reduce the sodium content, reduce or omit the milk used in this recipe, replacing it with sodium-free water.

Sugar-and-Spice Rice

This cinnamon-sugared creamy brown rice is topped with sweet, fresh berries.

Yield:	Prep time:	Cook time:	Serving size:
1 serving	3 minutes	5 minutes	1 bowl

Each serving has:		
350 calories	79 mg sodium	

1 cup cooked long-grain brown
  rice (about ⅓ cup uncooked)
½ cup fat-free milk
1 TB. firmly packed light brown
  sugar

¼ tsp. ground cinnamon
½ cup blackberries, raspberries,
  blueberries, or sliced
  strawberries

1. In a small saucepan over medium-high to high heat, stir together rice, milk, light brown sugar, and cinnamon. Bring to a boil. Immediately reduce heat to medium, and cook, stirring occasionally, for 3 or 4 minutes or until thick and creamy.

2. Spoon into a serving bowl, and let cool slightly. Add blackberries, stirring in as desired.

PINCH OF SAGE

If you have rice left over from last night's dinner, this breakfast is a delicious use for it. If you don't have leftover rice, substitute instant brown rice that cooks in 10 minutes. Remember that instant rices do contain a little sodium, from about 5 to 20 milligrams. Check the nutrition label.

Crunchy Berry Parfait

Fresh raspberries dressed in sweetened yogurt are joined by the crunch of granola, almonds, and coconut.

Yield:	Prep time:	Serving size:
1 serving	10 minutes	1 parfait

Each serving has:		
247 calories	86.2 mg sodium	

1 TB. sliced unsalted almonds	2 drops pure almond extract
1 TB. flaked coconut	½ cup granola
½ cup fat-free plain yogurt	⅔ cup fresh raspberries (or your
¾ tsp. confectioners' sugar	choice of other berries or fruit)

1. In a dry medium skillet over medium heat, toast almonds and coconut for 2 to 5 minutes. Shake the skillet often and watch carefully because they toast suddenly and can be quick to burn.

2. In a small bowl, stir together yogurt, confectioners' sugar, and almond extract.

3. In a tall parfait glass or other dessert dish, layer yogurt mixture, granola, and raspberries two or three times, as glass allows. Sprinkle toasted almonds and coconut on top.

SALT PITFALL

Granola, like many prepared foods, varies in sodium content from brand to brand. Read nutrition labels carefully.

Breakfast Banana Split

The classic banana, strawberry, and pineapple are served up with honey-sweetened yogurt all drizzled with chocolate and sprinkled with nuts.

Yield:	Prep time:	Serving size:
1 serving	2 minutes	1 dish
Each serving has:		
372.6 calories	105.9 mg sodium	

½ cup plain fat-free yogurt

2 tsp. honey

1 medium banana, peeled and split lengthwise

½ cup thinly sliced fresh strawberries

½ cup finely chopped fresh pineapple

1 tsp. chocolate syrup

1 TB. chopped unsalted dry-roasted peanuts

1. In a dessert dish or an oblong individual casserole dish, stir together yogurt and honey until blended.

2. Arrange banana halves along either long side of the dish. Spoon strawberries atop yogurt to the right side, and spoon pineapple atop yogurt to the left side.

3. Drizzle chocolate syrup over top. Sprinkle peanuts over all to serve.

Salternative: You can substitute frozen unsweetened sliced strawberries, thawed, and canned crushed pineapple, drained, for the fresh fruits in equal amounts. You also can substitute ½ cup of your favorite flavored yogurt for the plain yogurt and honey.

Breakfast Stir-Fry Scramble Pita

This pita breakfast sandwich encloses fluffy eggs enlivened with a bit of vegetables and peanut crunch.

Yield:	Prep time:	Cook time:	Serving size:
1 serving	3 minutes	3 minutes	1 pita pocket
Each serving has:			
303.4 calories	372.5 mg sodium		

2 large eggs

2 TB. cold water

¼ cup leftover Asian-Flavored Carrot Crunch Salsa (recipe in Chapter 13)

1 no-salt-added whole-wheat pita pocket

1. Heat a small skillet over medium heat, and coat with nonstick cooking spray.

2. In a small bowl, whisk eggs with water. Stir in Asian-Flavored Carrot Crunch Salsa, and cook for 3 minutes or until eggs are set.

3. Spoon into pita pocket to serve.

Salternative: The pita pocket allows you to eat this breakfast on the go. Of course, you can eat the eggs from a breakfast plate if you prefer.

Weekend Morning Indulgences

In This Chapter

- Enjoying unhurried weekend morning breakfast
- Cutting the sodium in breakfast foods
- Making brunch an event
- Serving breakfast—at dinner!

Leisurely weekend mornings provide time for relaxing, connecting with family, and indulging in flavorful breakfast foods. Although the goal of the weekday breakfast may be to get you going, weekend morning meals allow you to savor the flavor and the company.

With the recipes in this chapter, you'll find alternatives to some of the sodium explosion commonly found in leisurely breakfasts. Good ingredient choices can help, such as preparing your own sausage with ground turkey and spices. Sodium-conscious substitutions also play a role. Low-sodium cheeses, low-sodium breads, and sodium-free baking alternatives can bring breakfast back into reach.

Plus, you can easily accompany any of the dishes here with a selection of fresh fruits for a healthful, heartwarming gathering. So put the kettle on, set the breakfast table, and indulge!

Breakfast: Good *Any* Time

Leisurely breakfasts and the foods served are memorable because they only happen occasionally. When you have the time, use it to treat yourself and your loved ones to the eye-opening aromas and irresistible flavors of breakfast.

If your family prefers to lounge in bed on a Saturday morning, start cooking just before they normally awaken. The tantalizing smells wafting from the kitchen are sure to arouse them. If it's later than breakfast, call it brunch and enjoy it just the same.

You may also fill a lazy morning with extended family and friends. Serve a collection of dishes buffet style to make it easier on you if cooking for many people seems a daunting task. Most everyone loves brunch, and catching up with each other over enjoyable food is a great way to start the weekend.

Perhaps you just can't find the time for a long, luxurious weekend morning breakfast. Don't fret. You can serve these mouthwatering recipes just as easily for dinner any day of the week. Breakfast foods are simply wonderful, day or night.

PINCH OF SAGE

Sodium-free alternatives are available for baking powder and baking soda. You can use them to prepare your favorite pancakes, waffles, breakfast breads and muffins, and more. If you can't find Featherweight Baking Powder, Ener-G Baking Powder, or Ener-G Baking Soda near you, you can likely find some sources online. Simply enter the brand names into your favorite search engine and see what you can find.

Cinnamon Morning Apples

Delight in buttery sweet apple slices spiced with cinnamon and nutmeg.

Yield:	Prep time:	Cook time:	Serving size:
2 cups	5 minutes	16 minutes	½ cup
Each serving has:			
156.3 calories	1 mg sodium		

2 TB. unsalted butter

2 medium apples, peeled, cored, and cut into ½-in. slices

⅓ cup granulated sugar

½ tsp. ground cinnamon

Pinch ground nutmeg

1. In a medium nonstick skillet over low heat, melt butter. Add apples, sugar, cinnamon, and nutmeg, and stir to coat.

2. Increase heat to medium-low or medium, and sauté for 12 to 16 minutes or until apples are tender, stirring frequently to prevent sticking and scorching. Serve as a side dish or as a topping for pancakes, waffles, or French toast.

PINCH OF SAGE

If you need to slice the apples ahead of time, prevent browning by rubbing the apple slices with a slice of lemon. Try Braeburn, Golden Delicious, Granny Smith, or Jonagold apple varieties for this recipe.

Crisp Home Fries

Mildly spiced, these potatoes are crisp-browned alongside flavorful minced onion.

Yield:	Prep time:	Cook time:	Serving size:
1 cup	5 minutes	25 minutes	$\frac{1}{2}$ cup
Each serving has:			
167.4 calories	4 mg sodium		

1 TB. extra-virgin olive oil

2 medium all-purpose potatoes, scrubbed and diced

$\frac{1}{2}$ tsp. onion powder

$\frac{1}{2}$ tsp. garlic powder

$\frac{1}{4}$ tsp. chipotle chili powder or cayenne

$\frac{1}{4}$ tsp. freshly ground black pepper

1 TB. minced yellow onions

1. In a medium nonstick skillet over medium to medium-low heat, heat extra-virgin olive oil. Add potatoes, stir to coat evenly, and cook for 5 minutes, stirring frequently.

2. Add onion powder, garlic powder, chipotle chili powder, and pepper, and cook for 15 minutes, stirring frequently.

3. Stir in onions, reduce heat to low, and cook, stirring often, for 3 minutes or until onions are translucent and tender.

PINCH OF SAGE

You can increase this recipe to serve the number of people you have for breakfast. Just be sure to use a skillet large enough to keep the potatoes in a single layer. If your preference is for softer home fries or if you won't be available to stir the potatoes frequently, cook them slower and longer.

Eggless Potato Pancakes

Lightly seasoned lacy potato shreds are crisp-browned on the outside and tender on the inside.

Yield:	Prep time:	Cook time:	Serving size:
10 potato pancakes	8 minutes	10 minutes per batch	2 potato pancakes
Each serving has:			
73.1 calories	4 mg sodium		

2 medium-large all-purpose potatoes, scrubbed

$\frac{1}{2}$ medium yellow onion

1 TB. chopped fresh Italian parsley

$\frac{1}{4}$ tsp. freshly ground black pepper

$\frac{1}{8}$ tsp. garlic powder

1 TB. all-purpose flour

1. Grate potatoes and onion into a large bowl of cold water. Drain in a colander, and press out as much liquid as possible. Squeeze out remaining liquid with paper towels.

2. Place potato mixture in a large dry bowl. Add parsley, pepper, and garlic powder, and stir. Add flour, and stir well to combine.

3. Heat an extra-large nonstick skillet over medium heat, and coat with nonstick cooking spray.

4. For each pancake, spoon in about $\frac{1}{3}$ cup potato mixture without crowding the skillet, cooking in batches as necessary. Flatten each pancake with the back of a spatula, keeping in a single pile. Cook for 5 or 6 minutes or until browned on the underside, occasionally pressing down with a spatula as it cooks. Turn and cook the other side for 5 or 6 minutes or until golden-brown on the underside and potatoes are tender, pressing occasionally. Remove from the skillet and keep warm until all potato pancakes are done.

Salternative: For hash browns, melt about 1 tablespoon unsalted butter in the skillet. Add potato mixture all at once, and cook, stirring often, for 10 minutes or until potatoes are tender.

Lemon Raspberry Crepes

Thin, tender crepes wrap around tangy lemon yogurt and fresh raspberries and are then sweetened with a sprinkling of confectioners' sugar.

Yield:	Prep time:	Cook time:	Serving size:
14 crepes	25 minutes	15 minutes	2 crepes

Each serving has:		
143.2 calories	40 mg sodium	

2 large eggs

½ cup fat-free milk

½ cup water

1 cup all-purpose flour

2 TB. unsalted butter, melted

1 (6-oz.) container fat-free lemon yogurt

½ dry pt. fresh raspberries

2 tsp. confectioners' sugar

1. In a medium bowl, blend together eggs, milk, and water. Stir in flour and butter, and let batter stand for 20 minutes.

2. Coat an electric skillet generously with nonstick cooking spray, and preheat to 350°F.

3. Pour 2 tablespoons batter onto the hot skillet for each crepe, and cook for 30 seconds or until edges are dry and underside is golden. Turn and cook for 15 more seconds or until golden. Remove to a sheet of waxed paper, and repeat with remaining batter.

4. Spread yogurt down centers of crepes, and scatter raspberries over yogurt. Fold over sides of crepes, and lightly sprinkle tops with confectioners' sugar.

PINCH OF SAGE

These basic crepes don't have sugar in the batter, so you may fill them with your choice of savory fillings as well. See the recipe for Sautéed Spinach and Mushrooms Crepes in Chapter 8 for one idea.

Hearty Buckwheat Pancakes

Great grains pack these filling pancakes lightly sweetened with honey.

Yield:	Prep time:	Cook time:	Serving size:
10 pancakes	10 minutes	15 minutes	2 pancakes
Each serving has:			
252.4 calories	41.2 mg sodium		

½ cup whole-wheat flour	3 TB. extra-light olive oil
¼ cup buckwheat flour	2 TB. honey
¼ cup all-purpose flour	1 cup fat-free milk
¼ cup quick oats	1 large egg, beaten
3 tsp. *sodium-free* baking powder	

1. In a large bowl, combine whole-wheat flour, buckwheat flour, all-purpose flour, quick oats, and sodium-free baking powder. Add extra-light olive oil, honey, milk, and egg, and whisk together just until blended.

2. Heat a large, nonstick skillet over medium heat, and coat with nonstick cooking spray.

3. Pour ¼ cup batter into the skillet for each pancake, and cook until bubbly on top, just firm at edges, and golden on bottom. Turn and cook until golden on underside. Repeat with remaining batter.

DEFINITION

Sodium-free labeling is applied to foods that contain less than 5 milligrams sodium per serving. Sodium-free baking powder rises like regular baking powder without the high sodium content. (Read the label for any special instructions.)

Pumpkin-Spiced French Toast

The flavor of pumpkin pie coats the hearty *sprouted-grain bread* slices in this unique French toast.

Yield:	Prep time:	Cook time:	Serving size:
12 slices	5 minutes	8 minutes per batch	2 slices

Each serving has:			
223.5 calories	44.2 mg sodium		

3 large eggs, at room temperature	1 tsp. vanilla extract
1 cup canned pumpkin purée	1½ tsp. pumpkin pie spice
½ cup fat-free milk	12 slices sodium-free sprouted-grain bread

1. Heat an extra-large nonstick skillet over medium to medium-low heat, and coat with nonstick cooking spray.

2. In a large, shallow dish, whisk eggs until lemon-colored.

3. Add pumpkin purée, milk, and vanilla extract, and whisk until blended. Add pumpkin pie spice, and whisk until incorporated.

4. Place each bread slice, 1 at a time, in pumpkin mixture, turning to coat both sides. Transfer to the skillet, and cook for 4 minutes or until golden and cooked on the underside. Turn and cook for 4 minutes on the other side or until golden. Remove from the skillet and keep warm until all French toast is done. Serve by drizzling on pure maple syrup, dusting on confectioners' sugar, or topping with fruit as desired.

Salternative: If you prefer your French toast sweetened without toppings, stir 1 tablespoon or more granulated sugar into the pumpkin mixture.

DEFINITION

Sprouted-grain breads are made from freshly sprouted whole grains and, therefore, contain no flour. Loaves are typically found in your supermarket's freezer section, but not always. The Ezekiel 4:9 low-sodium version is sodium free.

Golden-Baked Pancake

This fluffy whole-wheat, oven-baked pancake is sweetened with cinnamon and sugar.

Yield:	Prep time:	Cook time:	Serving size:
1 (9-inch) pancake	10 minutes	20 minutes	$\frac{1}{6}$ pancake
Each serving has:			
259.1 calories	64.7 mg sodium		

$\frac{1}{3}$ cup unsalted butter	3 TB. granulated sugar
4 large eggs	$\frac{1}{2}$ tsp. ground cinnamon
1 cup fat-free milk	
1 cup whole-wheat flour	

1. Preheat the oven to 425°F.

2. Place butter in a 9-inch round cake pan, and melt it in the preheating oven.

3. In a blender, whip eggs and milk on high speed for 10 seconds or until blended. Add whole-wheat flour, and beat on high speed for 20 seconds or until thoroughly blended.

4. Remove bubbling butter from the oven. Pour batter into the hot pan, and sprinkle sugar and cinnamon over top.

5. Bake for 20 minutes or until raised and golden. Cut into 6 wedges. Serve with Cinnamon Morning Apples (recipe earlier in this chapter), drizzle on your favorite syrup, or dust with confectioners' sugar.

SALT PITFALL

Use caution when removing butter from the oven. It's hot and bubbling, and it can spatter.

Good-Start Sausage Patties

Traditional sausage herbs and spices season ground turkey crisp from the broiler.

Yield:	Prep time:	Cook time:	Serving size:
4 patties	10 minutes	13 minutes	1 patty

Each serving has:		
119.1 calories	74.1 mg sodium	

¼ tsp. plus ⅛ tsp. rubbed sage

¼ tsp. dried basil

¼ tsp. dried oregano

¼ tsp. freshly ground black pepper

¼ tsp. garlic powder

⅛ tsp. dried dill weed

⅛ tsp. ground allspice

⅛ tsp. ground nutmeg

Pinch Firehouse Chili Powder (recipe in Chapter 14) or other salt-free chili powder

2 TB. water

1 large egg white

¾ lb. ground turkey

1. Preheat the broiler to high. Spray the rack of a broiler pan with nonstick cooking spray.

2. In a medium bowl, combine sage, basil, oregano, pepper, garlic powder, dill weed, allspice, nutmeg, Firehouse Chili Powder, water, egg white, and ground turkey. Mix well.

3. Shape mixture into 4 (3-inch) patties. Arrange on the broiler rack.

4. Broil 3 or 4 inches from the heat source for 10 minutes. Turn patties over, rotate, and broil on the other side for 3 or 4 minutes or until a food thermometer into the center reads 165°F.

PINCH OF SAGE

The first time you try these breakfast patties, follow the recipe. Then, experiment with the seasonings until they taste just perfect to you.

Roasted Asparagus Frittata

Oven-roasted asparagus, mushrooms, garlic, and green onions flavor the smooth egg base topped with a touch of Swiss cheese.

Yield:	Prep time:	Cook time:	Serving size:
6 wedges	5 minutes	18 minutes	1 wedge

Each serving has:	
122.1 calories	74.2 mg sodium

1 cup 1-in. lengths fresh asparagus	6 large eggs
1 cup sliced button mushrooms	¼ tsp. garlic powder
1 medium green onion, chopped	¼ tsp. crushed red pepper flakes
1 medium clove garlic, minced	¼ cup low-sodium Swiss cheese
1 TB. extra-virgin olive oil	

1. Preheat the oven to 400°F.

2. On a medium nonstick baking sheet, combine asparagus, mushrooms, green onion, and garlic. Drizzle extra-virgin olive oil over all, and stir to coat evenly. Bake on the top oven shelf for 10 minutes or until asparagus is tender.

3. Meanwhile, in a medium bowl, whisk eggs until lemon-colored. Whisk in garlic powder and crushed red pepper flakes.

4. Heat a 10-inch ovenproof nonstick skillet over medium to medium-low heat. Add asparagus mixture, and spread over the bottom of the skillet evenly. Add egg mixture, and cook without stirring for 5 minutes or until egg mixture is set on the bottom.

5. Preheat the broiler to high. Adjust the oven shelf as needed so it's 4 inches from the heat source.

6. Broil *frittata* for 2 minutes or until top is set, puffed, and golden brown. Sprinkle Swiss cheese over top of frittata, and broil for 30 seconds or until cheese is golden, watching carefully. Cut into 6 wedges to serve.

DEFINITION

A **frittata** is a skillet-cooked mixture of eggs and other ingredients that isn't stirred but is cooked slowly and then either flipped or finished under the broiler. This Italian-style egg dish differs from a French-style omelet in that the other ingredients are cooked *in* the eggs and not used as a filling.

Sweet Curried Eggs

Sautéed sweet onions and apples are curried and then used to season tomato-sauced scrambled eggs.

Yield:	Prep time:	Cook time:	Serving size:
1½ cups	5 minutes	15 minutes	¾ cup

Each serving has:			
317.1 calories	130.8 mg sodium		

2 TB. unsalted butter

½ cup diced sweet onions

1 medium apple, cored and diced

½ tsp. salt-free curry powder

4 large eggs

¼ cup no-salt-added tomato sauce

1. In a medium nonstick skillet over medium heat, melt butter. Add sweet onions and apple, and sauté for 8 to 10 minutes or until tender. Stir in curry powder.

2. In a medium bowl, whisk eggs. Add tomato sauce, and whisk until blended. Pour into the skillet, and cook, stirring frequently, for 5 minutes or until eggs are set.

Veggie Confetti Frittata

Sautéed bell peppers and green onions mix with fresh tomatoes in golden-topped broiled eggs.

Yield:	Prep time:	Cook time:	Serving size:
1 frittata	5 minutes	10 minutes	1 frittata

Each serving has:	
168.2 calories	131.3 mg sodium

1 medium green onion, trimmed and thinly sliced

2 TB. finely diced red bell pepper

2 TB. finely diced green bell pepper

1 TB. cold water

2 large eggs

2 TB. finely diced tomatoes

1. Preheat the broiler to high. Generously spray an 8-inch ovenproof skillet with nonstick cooking spray. (If you don't have an ovenproof skillet, completely cover your skillet's plastic handle with foil. Remember when handling the skillet that the handle will be hot from the broiler.)

2. In the prepared skillet over medium-low heat, sauté green onion, red bell pepper, and green bell pepper for 3 minutes or until softened.

3. Meanwhile, in a small bowl, lightly beat cold water into eggs.

4. Stir tomatoes into the skillet, and arrange vegetable mixture in a single layer over the bottom of the skillet. Pour egg mixture into the skillet. Cook, without stirring, for 4 to 6 minutes or until eggs are *soft-set* on top.

5. Place the skillet under the broiler about 4 inches from the heat source. Broil for 1 minute or until top is golden brown.

Salternative: You may mix and match the sautéed ingredients in this frittata to suit individual tastes. Try mushrooms or sweet onions, or even add fresh herbs with the tomatoes. Prepare each diner's frittata to order.

DEFINITION

Soft-set refers to a stage when the eggs have started to firm, with some movement still, but they aren't set yet, in this case on the top.

Homemaker's Holiday Cranberry Coffeecake

Moist, mildly sweet coffeecake studded with fresh cranberries and walnuts is baked in a presentation-pretty fluted tube pan.

Yield:	Prep time:	Cook time:	Serving size:
1 fluted tube cake	20 minutes	50 minutes	1 slice ($\frac{1}{12}$ coffeecake)
Each serving has:			
458.4 calories	207.3 mg sodium		

2 cups whole-wheat flour

1 cup chopped cranberries, fresh or frozen

$1\frac{1}{4}$ cups chopped unsalted walnuts

1 cup unsalted butter, softened

2 cups granulated sugar

1 cup egg substitute

$\frac{1}{2}$ cup fat-free evaporated milk

$1\frac{1}{2}$ tsp. pure vanilla extract

1. Preheat the oven to 350°F. Generously spray a fluted tube pan with nonstick cooking spray with flour or with regular nonstick cooking spray and then lightly dust with flour.

2. In a medium mixing bowl, stir together whole-wheat flour, cranberries, and walnuts.

3. In a large mixing bowl, and using an electric mixer on medium speed, beat butter and sugar until light and fluffy. Add egg substitute $\frac{1}{4}$ cup at a time, mixing well after each addition. Stir in evaporated milk and vanilla extract, and mix well.

4. Add dry ingredients to wet ingredients, and blend just until moistened. Scrape batter into the prepared pan, and smooth top with a rubber spatula. Bake for 50 to 60 minutes or until a cake tester inserted in the center comes out clean.

PINCH OF SAGE

If you're not watching calories, you can drizzle on a confectioners' sugar glaze (just mix a very small amount of liquid, such as water or fruit juice, with confectioners' sugar). This coffeecake is pleasantly sweet without it, though, and has a texture much like a quick bread.

In the Lunchbox

At midday or whenever you want a lighter meal, a salad, soup, or sandwich—or any grouping of the three—can fill the bill. The combination of proteins, carbs, and vegetables or fruits keeps your diet well balanced and your stomach satisfied.

And with good food in your lunchbox, you decrease your risk of falling prey to fast-food drive-thru windows or the office vending machines and the often unhealthy and sodium-laden foods they offer.

Filling Lunchtime Salads

In This Chapter

* Eating healthfully from a single plate
* Sodium-smart salad fixings
* Shoring up your veggie servings
* To-go salads

Main-dish salads make fabulous lunches, and can do double-duty as light suppers or even healthful snacks in smaller portions. A single dish can encompass your protein, carb, veggie, and fruit needs. You can even add cooked meat, poultry, or fish to vegetable-based salads if you desire.

If you keep the sodium levels of your individual ingredients in mind, you can build a fantastic, mouthwatering salad that fits in your low-sodium dietary requirements. Plus, you'll naturally be eating a serving—or two, or three—of vegetables or fruits, helping you more easily meet the recommended daily intake ($2\frac{1}{2}$ cups vegetables and 2 cups fruit per day for a 2,000-calorie diet).

Delicious, easy to prepare, and packed with nutrients—let's do salads for lunch!

Healthful Fixings

Full-meal salads offer a great opportunity for making a meal meet all your food cravings. You can mix and match your favorite vegetables, fruits, meats, toppings, and salad dressings. You do have to be smart about which ingredients you choose, though, because some traditional salad fixings are high in sodium.

At a typical salad bar, you'll find many sodium pitfalls. Bacon bits, croutons, salted nuts and seeds, frozen peas, canned beans, pickled peppers, olives, cheeses, and commercially prepared salad dressings all threaten to blow your lo-so intentions. However, you can prepare sodium-sensible salads simply by substituting appropriate ingredients. Be certain any nuts or seeds you sprinkle on top of your salad are unsalted. Substitute no-salt-added canned peas and beans, or cook dried beans for even less sodium. Purchase any pickled items only if they're no-salt-added—same with olives. Opt for low-sodium cheeses.

And purchase—or prepare!—low-sodium salad dressings. (We give you several options in Chapter 6.) With sodium-smart ingredients, you can build a perfect salad.

Smart Salad Strategies

Making a main-dish salad part of your regular menu planning provides a wealth of benefits. Preparation is easy, and cooking, if any, is oftentimes quick. Indulging in a delicious salad each day makes it almost effortless to eat a wide variety of colorful veggies and fruits, giving your body a healthy dose of vitamins, minerals, antioxidants, and fiber. Plus, you can prepare and pack your salad to take a nutritious salad with you for lunch or a midday snack.

Packing a main-dish salad does require some savvy. You should always pour a salad dressing into a separate, covered container. Dressing the salad several hours before you plan on eating it results in wilted, droopy greens. If the dressing is mixed into the salad, such as for a chicken salad, transport the greens in a container separate from the salad. You can quickly reheat meats in the microwave if you like. Or you can enjoy the thoroughly cooked meats cold, as long as you've kept everything below 40°F. If you have access to a refrigerator, that's your best option. If not, use a cooler to maintain the freshness and safety of your meal.

PINCH OF SAGE

When tossing salads, try to include a rainbow of vegetables and fruits—reds, yellows, oranges, greens, blues, purples, and whites. The phytochemicals that provide the variety of colors also offer a wide range of healthful disease-deterring benefits—all without adding lots of calories or sodium.

Veggie-Packed Pasta Salad

Whole-wheat rotini is the vehicle for crunchy veggies and sweet peas in this classic Italian-dressed salad.

Yield:	Prep time:	Cook time:	Chill time:	Serving size:
6 cups	5 minutes	15 minutes	4 hours	1 cup

Each serving has:	
385.2 calories	4.6 mg sodium

8 oz. whole-wheat rotini pasta

1 medium tomato, cored, diced, and seeded as desired (about ½ cup)

¼ cup diced cucumber, seeded as desired

¼ cup diced yellow bell pepper

¼ cup drained, canned no-salt-added peas or lightly cooked fresh peas

1 cup Italian Dressing (recipe in Chapter 6) or other low-sodium Italian salad dressing

1. Cook pasta according to the package directions (omit salt). Drain and rinse under cold water.

2. In a large bowl, combine pasta, tomato, cucumber, yellow bell pepper, and peas.

3. Pour Italian Dressing over top, and stir to coat all. Cover and chill for at least 4 hours.

4. Stir again before serving.

PINCH OF SAGE

Use your favorite vegetables and beans in this salad—just keep the measurements the same. Choose a total of 1 cup vegetables, such as broccoli, cauliflower, zucchini, yellow squash, sweet onions, snow peas, and so on. Replace the peas with cooked dry beans or no-salt-added canned beans, such as kidney beans or chickpeas. You can even use your favorite low-sodium salad dressing. Serve it all on lettuce-lined salad plates for an attractive presentation.

Hearty Grilled Veggie Salad

Grilling imparts a smoky flavor to hearty veggies tossed with a sweet balsamic sauce.

Yield:	Prep time:	Cook time:	Serving size:
6 cups	40 minutes	25 minutes	1 cup

Each serving has:			
103.7 calories	13.1 mg sodium		

2 TB. extra-virgin olive oil

1 medium eggplant, cut into 1-in. slices

1 small zucchini, cut into 1-in. slices

1 medium summer squash, cut into 1-in. slices

1 small yellow onion, cut into 1-in. slices (do not separate rings)

1 medium red bell pepper, ribs and seeds removed, and cut into large wedges

1 lb. plum tomatoes, cored, seeded if desired, and quartered lengthwise

2 medium cloves garlic, minced

2 TB. chopped fresh basil

2 TB. balsamic vinegar

¼ tsp. freshly ground black pepper

1. Preheat a double-sided indoor grill.

2. Lightly rub extra-virgin olive oil over cut sides of eggplant, zucchini, summer squash, and onion. Add veggies to the grill and cook for 3 to 5 minutes or until fork-tender.

3. Add bell pepper, and cook for 10 minutes or until tender.

4. Add tomatoes, and cook for 2 minutes or until just charred.

5. Remove vegetables to a large cutting board, and chop, peeling tomatoes as desired.

6. In a large bowl, combine vegetables, garlic, basil, balsamic vinegar, and pepper, and stir to coat. Let stand for at least 30 minutes. Stir again before serving warm or at room temperature. Serve vegetable mixture over mixed salad greens, if you like.

Salternative: The intense flavor of grilling is delicious, but if you feel this salad needs spiced up a bit, shake on a garlic-and-herb salt-substitute seasoning blend.

PINCH OF SAGE

Grill these vegetables outdoors, if you prefer. You may want to slice the eggplant, zucchini, and squash lengthwise to keep them safely atop the grilling rack. Grill the tomatoes whole and the onion and bell pepper halved so they don't slip through the grate. Or place the vegetables in a nonstick grilling basket, if you have one.

Wild Turkey Salad

The nutty taste of wild rice complements sweet and savory turkey bites.

Yield:	Prep time:	Serving size:
4 servings	10 minutes	½ cup lettuce with 1 cup turkey salad

Each serving has:		
247.7 calories	49.4 mg sodium	

2 cups cooked wild rice

1 cup finely cubed cooked turkey breast

1 cup halved seedless red grapes

1 cup skin-on diced apples

¼ cup finely diced red bell pepper

¼ cup chopped unsalted walnuts

½ cup fat-free plain yogurt

4 tsp. fresh lime juice

4 tsp. chopped fresh parsley

2 cups torn green-leaf lettuce, lightly packed

1. In a medium bowl, combine wild rice, turkey, grapes, apples, bell pepper, and walnuts.

2. In another small bowl, stir together yogurt, lime juice, and parsley. Add to rice mixture, and stir until evenly coated.

3. To serve, line each of 4 plates with ½ cup lettuce, and mound 1 cup salad on top.

SALT PITFALL

Wild rice—which is not really a rice at all, but an aquatic grass—can be found near the many boxes of convenience rice mixes on your grocer's shelf. Take care not to pick up a package of wild rice with a high-sodium seasoning packet included. Purchase plain wild rice, which is usually sold in a smaller box.

Lemon-Kissed Tuna-Stuffed Tomatoes

Albacore tuna is brightened by a citrusy squeeze of lemon juice and fresh add-ins and served in a tomato cup.

Yield:	Prep time:	Cook time:	Serving size:
2 stuffed tomatoes	10 minutes	3 minutes	1 stuffed tomato

Each serving has:			
154.7 calories	64 mg sodium		

2 TB. fresh lemon juice

2 medium green onions, chopped

2 TB. diced red bell pepper

1 TB. chopped fresh parsley

1 (6-oz.) can *very low-sodium* albacore tuna packed in water, drained

3 TB. fat-free plain yogurt

2 medium tomatoes, cored

1. In a nonstick medium skillet over medium heat, heat lemon juice just until hot. Add green onions, red bell pepper, and parsley, and cook for 1 or 2 minutes or until softened.

2. Add tuna, flaking with a fork. Cook for 1 or 2 minutes or until heated through, and remove from heat. Stir in yogurt, evenly coating tuna and vegetables.

3. To serve, slice tomatoes into 8 wedges each beginning at the cored top without cutting through bottoms of tomatoes. Divide tuna mixture between sliced tomatoes.

Salternative: You can easily double this recipe as needed.

DEFINITION

Very low-sodium is used on product labels to identify foods that contain no more than 35 milligrams sodium per serving.

Golden Chicken Tenders Salad

Crunchy and fresh, these salad favorites are drizzled with a creamy, garlicky dressing.

Yield:	Prep time:	Cook time:	Serving size:
4 servings	10 minutes	6 minutes	1 cup greens with 4 ounces chicken, $\frac{1}{4}$ additions, and 2 tablespoons salad dressing

Each serving has:	
323.3 calories	75.9 mg sodium

2 tsp. fresh lemon juice

1 lb. chicken tenders, rinsed and patted dry with paper towels

$\frac{1}{2}$ tsp. salt-free poultry seasoning

4 cups packed torn salad greens

2 small tomatoes, cored and cut into thin wedges

$\frac{1}{2}$ small green bell pepper, ribs and seeds removed, and cut into thin strips

$\frac{1}{2}$ small yellow bell pepper, ribs and seeds removed, and cut into thin strips

$\frac{1}{2}$ medium red onion, thinly sliced

4 medium button mushrooms, wiped with a damp paper towel, trimmed, and sliced

3 TB. sliced unsalted almonds

1 TB. unsalted sunflower seed kernels

$\frac{1}{2}$ cup Golden Garlic Dressing (recipe in Chapter 6)

1. Preheat a double-sided indoor grill.

2. Drizzle lemon juice over chicken tenders, and season with poultry seasoning. Add chicken to the grill, and cook, in batches, for 3 minutes or until done.

3. Serve chicken on a bed of salad greens with tomatoes, green bell pepper, yellow bell pepper, red onion, mushrooms, almonds, and sunflower seed kernels. Drizzle Golden Garlic Dressing over all.

SALT PITFALL

Make this salad your own with your favorite vegetables, salad toppings, and salad dressing. But keep in mind that many traditional salad additions are higher in sodium, including bacon bits, frozen peas, canned beans, cheeses, and commercial salad dressings. You may have to forego some of your old favorites or choose sodium-smart substitutes, such as homemade salad dressings, cooked dried beans, and low-sodium cheeses.

Lightly Curried Fruit and Chicken Salad

Tangy lemon yogurt coats tropical fruits and berries paired with meaty chicken atop mixed greens.

Yield:	Prep time:	Cook time:	Serving size:
4 servings	10 minutes	2 minutes	1 cup greens with 1¼ cups chicken salad

Each serving has:		
339.6 calories	91.4 mg sodium	

2 cups diced cooked chicken breast	½ cup fresh red raspberries
1 tsp. fresh lemon juice	⅛ tsp. salt-free curry powder or more to taste
½ cup sliced unsalted almonds	½ cup fat-free, sugar-free lemon yogurt
1 medium papaya, peeled, seeded, and cubed	4 cups packed spring mix salad greens
1 large banana, peeled and thinly sliced	
½ cup fresh blueberries	

1. Place chicken in a large bowl, and drizzle with lemon juice.

2. In a small dry skillet over medium heat, toast almonds for 2 to 5 minutes, watching carefully and shaking occasionally to keep from burning. Cool slightly.

3. Add almonds, papaya, banana, blueberries, and raspberries to chicken mixture, and stir.

4. In a small bowl, stir curry powder into yogurt until evenly distributed. Spoon into chicken mixture, and toss lightly until evenly coated.

5. Place 1 cup salad greens on each of 4 plates, mound 1¼ cups chicken mixture on top, and serve.

SALT PITFALL

Be certain your chicken was not seasoned with salt or other high-sodium seasonings or sauces when it was cooked. As long as the chicken hasn't been prepared with high-sodium seasonings, leftover chicken makes this recipe convenient and quick.

Chinese Chicken Salad

Crunchy Asian vegetables shine in a sweet pineapple dressing with juicy chicken strips.

Yield:	Prep time:	Marinate time:	Cook time:	Serving size:
2 servings	5 minutes	30 minutes	10 minutes	1¼ cups salad with ½ of chicken

Each serving has:	
248.6 calories	93.7 mg sodium

1 cup shredded napa cabbage

½ cup julienned carrots

½ cup julienned red bell peppers

½ cup julienned snow peas

¼ cup julienned green onions

¼ cup Asian Sweet Sesame Dressing (recipe in Chapter 6)

½ lb. chicken breast(s)

2 TB. pineapple juice, or less as needed

½ cup drained mandarin orange sections, fresh or canned

1 tsp. toasted sesame seeds

1. In a large bowl, combine napa cabbage, carrots, red bell peppers, snow peas, and green onions. Pour Asian Sweet Sesame Dressing over all, and toss to coat evenly. Cover and refrigerate for 30 minutes.

2. Meanwhile, in a medium nonstick skillet over medium to medium-high heat, sear chicken breast(s) for 2 minutes. Turn and sear the other side(s) for 2 minutes.

3. Slowly pour pineapple juice over top(s) of chicken, using just enough to coat (sugars will caramelize on the outside). Cover and cook for 6 to 8 minutes or until a food thermometer inserted into the center reads 170°F. Remove chicken to a cutting board, and let stand for 5 minutes before slicing into thin strips.

4. Add mandarin orange sections and sesame seeds to marinated salad, and toss well. Arrange chicken strips atop salad, and serve.

SALT PITFALL

Be careful when pouring the pineapple juice over the chicken breast(s). If you pour it all at once or pour in too much, the juice will just burn on the bottom of your skillet.

Spring Salmon Salad

The delicate, seasonal flavor of asparagus and peas pairs nicely with the charbroiled flavor of salmon.

Yield:	Prep time:	Cook time:	Serving size:
2 servings	15 minutes	10 minutes	1¼ cups greens with 3 ounces salmon, ½ additions, and 2 tablespoons vinaigrette

Each serving has:	
424.8 calories	102.5 mg sodium

6 oz. skin-on salmon

2 cups packed torn red-leaf lettuce, rinsed and patted dry

½ cup packed baby spinach leaves, stemmed and rinsed

½ cup steamed 1-in. asparagus pieces

½ small red onion, sliced

½ yellow bell pepper, ribs and seeds removed, and cut into thin strips

¼ cup drained no-salt-added canned peas or lightly cooked fresh peas

1 large hard-boiled egg, peeled and chopped

1 large tomato, cored and chopped

1 medium green onion, chopped

¼ cup Balsamic Vinaigrette (recipe in Chapter 6)

1. Preheat the broiler to high. Spray the rack of a broiler pan with nonstick cooking spray.

2. Place salmon on the broiler rack, and broil 4 to 6 inches from heat for 10 minutes per inch of thickness or until done.

3. Place lettuce and spinach onto 2 plates. Flake salmon over top. Add asparagus, red onion, bell pepper, peas, egg, tomato, and green onion. Drizzle on Balsamic Vinaigrette, and serve.

Salternative: You can double this recipe as needed.

PINCH OF SAGE

To hard-boil eggs, place eggs in a saucepan and cover with cold water. Cover the saucepan, and bring the water to a boil over high heat. When boiling, remove the pan from the heat. Let eggs stand, covered, for 20 minutes. Immediately rinse eggs under cold water until cooled, and leave them immersed in cold water as you peel them. This method will keep the surface of the yolks from developing a green cast (as does not using fresh eggs for hard-boiling). If you do find a green yolk or two, don't worry. They're perfectly safe to eat.

Pittsburgh Steak Salad

The steel city offers a hearty salad with seasoned steak and classic salad fixings all topped with the taste-twist of crisp fries.

Yield:	Prep time:	Marinate time:	Cook time:	Serving size:
2 servings	15 minutes	8 hours	4 minutes	1 cup greens with 4 ounces steak, ½ additions, and 2 tablespoons salad dressing

Each serving has:	
895.5 calories	139.6 mg sodium

¼ cup plus 2 tsp. extra-virgin olive oil

¼ cup red wine vinegar

2 medium cloves garlic, minced

1 tsp. ground black pepper

½ lb. thin sandwich steak

2 cups torn salad greens, lightly packed

1 medium tomato, cored, seeded if desired, and chopped

¼ medium cucumber, peeled and sliced

¼ cup shredded carrots

¼ cup shredded red cabbage

1 hard-boiled egg, chopped

¼ cup shredded low-sodium cheddar cheese

2 doz. Oven-Crisped Fries (recipe in Chapter 21)

¼ cup Sweet Onion Dressing (recipe in Chapter 6) or other favorite low-sodium salad dressing

1. In a large zipper-lock bag, combine ¼ cup extra-virgin olive oil, red wine vinegar, garlic, and pepper. Add steak. Seal the bag, and marinate in the refrigerator for 8 hours or overnight.

2. Remove steak from marinade, and discard marinade. Slice steak into 2-inch-wide strips.

3. In a large, nonstick skillet over medium heat, heat remaining 2 teaspoons extra-virgin olive oil. Add steak, and cook for 2 minutes. Turn and cook for 1 minute on other side or until done. Drain on a paper towel–lined plate.

4. Line each of 2 plates with 1 cup salad greens. Top with tomato, cucumber, carrots, red cabbage, egg, cheddar cheese, and Oven-Crisped Fries. Add steak, and drizzle Sweet Onion Dressing over all.

Salternative: If you've forgotten to marinate steak beforehand, cut it into strips and season it with ¼ teaspoon each ground black pepper, garlic powder, and onion powder, and cook as directed. You'll have a fast-fix lunch with great taste. If you can't find thin sandwich steak, you can substitute your favorite skillet steak cut. Just be certain to cook it as needed. The recipe can also be doubled.

SALT PITFALL

Discard any uncooked marinade because it has been in contact with raw meat and is likely to harbor illness-causing bacteria. If a recipe calls for using the marinade, be sure to bring it to a boil first.

Tex-Mex Chicken Fajita Salad

A skillet-sizzled medley with bell peppers, corn, and chicken warm up the cool condiments for a Southwestern taste trip.

Yield:	Prep time:	Marinate time:	Cook time:	Serving size:
4 servings	10 minutes	up to 4 hours	15 minutes	1 cup salad greens with 4 ounces chicken and $\frac{1}{4}$ additions

Each serving has:	
393.1 calories	177.2 mg sodium

Juice of 2 large limes

2 medium green onions, trimmed and sliced

3 medium cloves garlic, minced

3 TB. extra-virgin olive oil

1 TB. dried cilantro or 3 TB. chopped fresh cilantro

$\frac{1}{2}$ tsp. crushed red pepper flakes

$\frac{1}{4}$ tsp. ground coriander

$\frac{1}{4}$ tsp. anise seeds

1 lb. thin-sliced, boneless, skinless chicken breast, rinsed and patted dry on paper towels

$\frac{1}{2}$ large green bell pepper, ribs and seeds removed, and cut into thin strips

$\frac{1}{2}$ large red bell pepper, ribs and seeds removed, and cut into thin strips

1 medium yellow onion, halved and sliced

$\frac{1}{2}$ cup frozen whole-kernel corn, thawed

$\frac{1}{2}$ cup no-salt-added black beans, drained and rinsed

4 cups torn salad greens, lightly packed

$\frac{1}{2}$ cup coarsely crushed unsalted baked tortilla chips

1 cup Fresh-Taste Tomato Salsa (recipe in Chapter 13) or other low-sodium salsa

$\frac{1}{2}$ cup Great Guacamole (recipe in Chapter 10) or other low-sodium guacamole

$\frac{1}{2}$ cup fat-free sour cream

1. In a large zipper-lock bag, combine lime juice, green onions, garlic, 2 tablespoons extra-virgin olive oil, cilantro, crushed red pepper flakes, coriander, and anise seeds. Add chicken. Seal the bag, and marinate in the refrigerator for 4 hours, turning occasionally.

2. In a large, nonstick skillet over medium heat, heat remaining 1 tablespoon extra-virgin olive oil. Add green bell pepper, red bell pepper, and yellow onion, and sauté for 8 minutes or until onion is golden and bell peppers are tender. Remove to a medium bowl. Stir in corn and black beans.

3. Remove chicken from marinade, and discard marinade. Cut chicken into large strips. Add to the skillet over medium heat, and cook for 2 minutes on each side or until done. Remove to a paper towel–lined plate.

4. To assemble, line each of 4 plates with 1 cup salad greens. Top with chicken, bell pepper mixture, and tortilla chips. Add dollops of Fresh-Taste Tomato Salsa, Great Guacamole, and sour cream.

PINCH OF SAGE

If you can't find thin-sliced chicken breast, substitute regular boneless, skinless chicken breast. Cut it into strips, and cook until no pink remains and a thermometer inserted in the center reads 170°F.

Mexican Night Taco Salad

Spiced ground beef and all your favorite south-of-the-border flavors are served up on a plate.

Yield:	Prep time:	Cook time:	Serving size:
4 servings	10 minutes	10 minutes	1 salad

Each serving has:			
537.9 calories	264.2 mg sodium		

1 lb. 85-percent-lean ground beef

1½ tsp. Taco Seasoning Mix (recipe in Chapter 14)

4 doz. unsalted baked tortilla chips

4 cups torn salad greens, lightly packed

½ cup diced yellow onions

½ cup sliced black olives or no-salt-added sliced black olives

½ cup finely shredded low-sodium cheddar cheese

½ cup Fresh-Taste Tomato Salsa (recipe in Chapter 13) or other low-sodium salsa

½ cup Great Guacamole (recipe in Chapter 10) or other low-sodium guacamole

½ cup fat-free sour cream

1. In a large, nonstick skillet over medium heat, brown ground beef with Taco Seasoning Mix. Cook for 7 or 8 minutes or until browned and a thermometer inserted into the center of a piece of meat measures 160°F, stirring to break up meat. Remove with a slotted spoon to a paper towel–lined plate.

2. Line each of 4 plates with 12 tortilla chips. Spoon on ground beef mixture. Layer salad greens, onions, black olives, and cheddar cheese over top.

3. Add dollops of Fresh-Taste Tomato Salsa, Great Guacamole, and sour cream.

Salternative: Save on a bit of sodium by substituting low-sodium black olives, which have about 8 milligrams sodium per olive.

PINCH OF SAGE

This recipe calls for 85-percent-lean ground beef. If your doctor or nutritionist has indicated that you should watch your saturated fat intake, use a leaner cut. Ground turkey breast also works.

Jerk Shrimp Fruit-Studded Salad

Hot and spicy shrimp are cooled by the bites of fresh fruits in a sweet balsamic dressing.

Yield:	Prep time:	Cook time:	Serving size:
4 servings	8 minutes	3 minutes	1 salad
Each serving has:			
342.7 calories	289.2 mg sodium		

12 oz. large tail-off shrimp (about 25), peeled and deveined, and thawed (if using frozen)

1 TB. Jerk Seasoning Blend (recipe in Chapter 14)

6 cups torn mixed salad greens, lightly packed

2 cups hulled and halved fresh strawberries

1 cup fresh pineapple chunks

1 cup halved seedless green grapes

1 recipe Lemon-Pepper Balsamic Dressing (recipe in Chapter 6)

1. Preheat the broiler to high. Coat the rack of a broiler pan with nonstick cooking spray.

2. Pat shrimp dry with paper towels and place in a zipper-lock bag. Add Jerk Seasoning Blend, close bag, and shake well to coat all shrimp evenly. Arrange shrimp on the broiler rack, and broil 4 inches from the heat source for 3 minutes or until opaque throughout.

3. On individual serving plates, evenly divide mixed salad greens, strawberries, pineapple chunks, green grapes, and shrimp. Drizzle Lemon-Pepper Balsamic Dressing over all. Serve immediately.

 SALT PITFALL

Frozen shrimp are processed with salt and sodium tripolyphosphate so you'll want to check the nutrition labels carefully to choose the brand with the least sodium per serving. Pick fresh shrimp if you need a lower-sodium option.

Super Salad Dressings

In This Chapter

- Nixing the high-sodium bottled dressings
- Easy homemade salad dressings
- Enjoying the natural taste of freshly made dressings
- Using discretion with dressings

Salad dressing can make a good salad even better! A flavorful dressing can complement the salad ingredients and bring out their crisp, fresh taste. With just the right balance of a delightful salad dressing, a bowlful of greens transforms into a delicious endeavor.

Perhaps you're thinking: *Sure, I love salad dressings, so why are you torturing me with how great-tasting they are? I can't have bottled salad dressings now that I'm watching my sodium intake.* Hogwash! You can prepare a plethora of luscious dressings with little effort or fanfare. Salad dressing doesn't come from a bottle any more than bacon comes from a frying pan. With homemade salad dressings, you can go hog wild again!

Fast, Fresh, and Fabulous

If you enjoy your green salads without a dressing, you don't have to concern yourself with the high sodium content of most bottled salad dressings. The same goes for tried-and-true vinegar-and-oil purists. However, if you love richly dressed greens, you may be heartbroken to discover the amount of sodium in a single serving of your favorite bottled dressing. If you've just got to have your salad dressing, a selection of sodium-free varieties are available.

Better yet, you can whip up your own fast, fresh, and fabulous salad dressings right in your own kitchen. You only need a few ingredients, a small bowl, and a whisk or a blender, and *voilà!* You've created the perfect salad dressing to complement the salad you're ready to eat right now. If you have 5 to 10 minutes, you can take a naked green salad and dress it up in style.

We've included a wide range of recipes here to cover an array of individual tastes, as well as any individual's taste on any given day. So whether you're a Balsamic Vinaigrette regular or a daily dressing swinger, you'll find a dressing you'll like here. Plus, we've included a flavorsome dressing for potato and macaroni salads, as well as a creamy dressing for fruit salads. All the dressings in this chapter are fresh and as bright-tasting as your lovingly selected salad fixings.

PINCH OF SAGE

Whenever a recipe indicates that you should whisk dressing ingredients until blended, you can opt to combine the ingredients in a jar with a tight-fitting lid; instead of whisking, shake well until combined. Can cooking get any easier?

A Note on Oil

The salad dressing recipes in this chapter call for extra-virgin olive oil when needed. You can, of course, substitute your favorite oils or even experiment with subtle taste differences when employing different oils.

We've suggested olive oil because the Food and Drug Administration now allows olive oil labels to claim …

> Limited and not conclusive scientific evidence suggests that eating about 2 tablespoons (23 grams) of olive oil daily may reduce the risk of coronary heart disease due to the monounsaturated fat in olive oil. To achieve this possible benefit, olive oil is to replace a similar amount of saturated fat and not increase the total number of calories you eat in a day.

So you can help your heart health and enjoy a delicious dressing at the same time. Can't beat that!

Getting Caught in a Downpour

You have a big, beautiful salad in front of you, full of crisp greens, a rainbow of veggies and maybe fruits, unsalted nuts or seeds, and numerous nutritional benefits. It's time to add the dressing—but wait! Now is the time to show some constraint. Don't succumb to the temptation to drown those poor greens. You don't need a soggy salad.

Most of the following dressings have a 2-tablespoon serving size. This amount is sufficient for a large salad, so if you're eating a small side salad with your meal, cut back the dressing to about 1 tablespoon or less. You should always use just enough dressing to make the taste of your salad pop and not any more.

If you're prone to using too much dressing, there is help. Some folks find it helpful to precisely measure. Knowing how much you're consuming is always a good idea, especially if you're not good at eyeballing the amount. (You can test your accuracy, if you like. Pour the amount of dressing you would normally drizzle over your salad and then measure it. And don't be surprised if it measures a bit more than you thought.)

Another method that may help you control your portions is lightly dipping each forkful into a small container of measured salad dressing. Each bite has the perfect complement of dressing, and you won't eat a drop more than your salad requires.

You could also dress and toss a salad and not serve dressing separately. After you assemble all your ingredients and add a small amount of dressing, toss it well to evenly coat the salad fixings. You'll get great taste without the puddle of surplus salad dressing at the bottom of the bowl.

Armed with a plan, you can dress up your favorite salads with great, complementary salad dressings and say bye-bye to bottles of sodium-laden salad dressings and hello to easy, homemade yum!

Asian Sweet Sesame Dressing

The sweetness of pineapple juice carries the classic Asian flavors of sesame, ginger, and cilantro.

Yield:	Prep time:	Serving size:
$\frac{1}{2}$ cup	3 minutes	2 tablespoons

Each serving has:		
41.3 calories	0 mg sodium	

3 TB. unsweetened pineapple juice

3 TB. sodium-free rice vinegar

1 TB. dark sesame seed oil

$\frac{1}{2}$ TB. grated fresh gingerroot

$\frac{1}{2}$ TB. chopped fresh cilantro

1. In a small bowl, combine pineapple juice, rice vinegar, and sesame seed oil. Whisk until well blended.

2. Add gingerroot and cilantro, and whisk to blend. Refrigerate any leftovers tightly covered for up to 2 days.

PINCH OF SAGE

Look for dark amber–colored sesame seed oil in your supermarket's Asian food section. This fragrant oil is used for flavoring, and a little goes a long way.

Garlic-Pepper Croutons

What's a salad without croutons? Satisfy your craving for a crisp crunch with these spicy salad toppers. They're also delicious as soup toppers!

Yield:	Prep time:	Cook time:	Serving size:
2½ cups	5 minutes	20 minutes	¼ cup

Each serving has:	
50 calories	0 mg sodium

3 cups (¾-in.-cubed) sodium-free sprouted-grain bread

2 TB. extra-virgin olive oil

½ tsp. garlic powder

½ tsp. freshly ground black pepper

¼ tsp. onion powder

1. Preheat the oven to 350°F.

2. Place bread cubes in a large, shallow dish. Drizzle extra-virgin olive oil evenly over bread cubes, and sprinkle garlic powder, pepper, and onion powder over top. Using 2 forks, toss gently to coat bread cubes evenly.

3. Transfer bread cubes to a large nonstick baking sheet, and arrange in a single layer. Bake for 10 minutes or until browned and aromatic. Stir well and bake for 10 more minutes or until well toasted.

4. Cool croutons before storing in the refrigerator in an airtight container for up to 2 weeks.

PINCH OF SAGE

Oils can become rancid with age or improper storage. To get the most out of your oils' shelf life, store tightly covered in a cool, dark place—and not next to the stove. When using, keep the oils away from light exposure as much as possible. Buy oils in opaque containers when available.

Vinegar-and-Oil French Dressing

This smooth and simple dressing is flavored with mild paprika.

Yield:	Prep time:	Chill time:	Serving size:
1⅛ cups	5 minutes	30 minutes	2 tablespoons
Each serving has:			
160.9 calories	0.1 mg sodium		

¾ cup extra-virgin olive oil

3 TB. fresh lemon juice

3 TB. white vinegar

½ tsp. paprika

¼ tsp. ground white pepper

1. In a small bowl, whisk together extra-virgin olive oil, lemon juice, white vinegar, paprika, and white pepper until thoroughly blended.

2. Cover and chill for at least 30 minutes to allow flavors to mingle. Whisk again before serving. Refrigerate any leftovers tightly covered for up to 2 weeks.

Salternative: To make **All-Thyme-Favorite French Dressing,** add ½ teaspoon dried thyme to this recipe.

Italian Dressing

Oregano and basil flavor the classic vinegar and olive oil dressing.

Yield:	Prep time:	Serving size:
1 cup	5 minutes	2 tablespoons
Each serving has:		
183.2 calories	0.2 mg sodium	

¾ cup extra-virgin olive oil

¼ cup white vinegar

1 tsp. granulated sugar

¼ tsp. dried oregano

¼ tsp. dried basil

¼ tsp. onion powder

¼ tsp. garlic powder

¼ tsp. Salt-Shaker Substitute (recipe in Chapter 14)

⅛ tsp. freshly ground black pepper

1. In a small bowl, combine extra-virgin olive oil, white vinegar, sugar, oregano, basil, onion powder, garlic powder, Salt-Shaker Substitute, and pepper. Whisk until thoroughly blended.

2. Whisk again before serving. Refrigerate any leftovers tightly covered for up to 2 weeks.

PINCH OF SAGE

You may use another savory salt-free salt-substitute seasoning blend if you prefer. You can't omit it altogether, though, because you'll lose a certain depth of flavor.

Sweet Onion Dressing

Savory salads are well dressed with the sweet smack of mild onions this dressing brings.

Yield:	Prep time:	Serving size:
1 cup	5 minutes	2 tablespoons
Each serving has:		
101.2 calories	0.3 mg sodium	

6 TB. extra-virgin olive oil

4 TB. white vinegar

¼ large sweet onion, coarsely chopped

1 small clove garlic

4 tsp. granulated sugar

¼ tsp. ground dry mustard

¾ tsp. Salt-Shaker Substitute (recipe in Chapter 14) or other salt-free salt-substitute seasoning blend

1. In a blender, place extra-virgin olive oil, white vinegar, onion, garlic, sugar, dry mustard, and Salt-Shaker Substitute.

2. Blend on high speed for 10 to 15 seconds or until smooth. Refrigerate any leftovers tightly covered for up to 2 weeks.

PINCH OF SAGE

To peel a garlic clove easily, smash it under a wide knife blade, such as that of a chef's knife (the blade facing away from you, of course). The papery peel should slough off. Cut off and discard the woody root end.

Red Wine Ginger Dressing

The kick of ginger enhances the bite of red wine vinegar in this zippy dressing.

Yield:	Prep time:	Serving size:
1⅜ cups	10 minutes	2 tablespoons
Each serving has:		
143.2 calories	0.7 mg sodium	

¾ cup plus 1 TB. extra-virgin olive oil	4 medium cloves garlic, minced
½ cup red wine vinegar	1 tsp. ground ginger
	¼ tsp. freshly ground black pepper

1. In a small bowl, combine extra-virgin olive oil, red wine vinegar, garlic, ginger, and pepper.

2. Whisk until thoroughly blended. Refrigerate any leftovers tightly covered for up to 2 weeks.

Salternative: Reduce the amount of red wine vinegar if you don't care for the tangy taste.

Balsamic Vinaigrette

Sweeter than other vinegars, balsamic vinegar lends to a smooth-flavored vinaigrette deepened by simple spice enhancers.

Yield:	Prep time:	Serving size:
⅜ cup	10 minutes	2 tablespoons
Each serving has:		
177.2 calories	2.9 mg sodium	

¼ cup extra-virgin olive oil	¾ tsp. granulated sugar
2 TB. balsamic vinegar	⅛ tsp. Salt-Shaker Substitute (recipe in Chapter 14)
1 tsp. ground dry mustard	⅛ tsp. freshly ground black pepper
1 medium clove garlic, minced	

1. In a small bowl, combine extra-virgin olive oil, balsamic vinegar, dry mustard, garlic, sugar, Salt-Shaker Substitute, and pepper.

2. Whisk until thoroughly blended. Refrigerate any leftovers tightly covered for up to 2 weeks. Mix well before serving.

PINCH OF SAGE

Adjust this recipe for the amount you need, but don't mix up too much. Homemade dressings don't have the shelf life of commercial brands. They're measured in days and weeks instead of months. But they do have a fresh, superior flavor.

Citrus-Kissed Dressing

Orange, lemon, and lime juices balance the olive oil in this smooth, honey-sweetened dressing.

Yield:	Prep time:	Serving size:
4 cups	10 minutes	2 tablespoons
Each serving has:		
198.2 calories	5.2 mg sodium	

2 cups extra-virgin olive oil

¾ cup granulated sugar

1 cup fresh orange juice

¼ cup fresh lemon juice

3 TB. fresh lime juice

1 large pasteurized egg

1 large pasteurized egg white

2 TB. honey

1. In a blender, combine extra-virgin olive oil, sugar, orange juice, lemon juice, lime juice, pasteurized egg, pasteurized egg white, and honey.

2. Blend for 30 seconds or until well blended. Refrigerate any leftovers tightly covered for 1 or 2 days.

PINCH OF SAGE

You must use pasteurized eggs in this recipe because it's uncooked. Regular eggs—even fresh, uncracked ones—leave you susceptible to food-borne illness. Look for egg cartons labeled pasteurized in the refrigerated case where you find regular eggs.

Lemon-Pepper Balsamic Dressing

This sweet balsamic vinaigrette flavored with a sharp touch of lemon and pepper dresses a savory salad deliciously.

Yield:	Prep time:	Serving size:
½ cup	5 minutes	2 tablespoons
Each serving has:		
142.7 calories	5.2 mg sodium	

¼ cup extra-virgin olive oil

¼ cup balsamic vinegar

1 TB. firmly packed light brown sugar

½ TB. fresh lemon juice

⅛ tsp. dried lemon peel

⅛ tsp. freshly ground black pepper

1. In a small bowl, combine extra-virgin olive oil, balsamic vinegar, light brown sugar, lemon juice, lemon peel, and pepper.

2. Whisk until well blended. Refrigerate any leftovers tightly covered for up to 2 weeks.

Salternative: Substitute regular white vinegar for the balsamic vinegar for an equally tasty salad dressing.

Creamy Avocado Dressing

The succulent mouthfeel of ripe avocado with a splash of lime comes through in this thick dressing.

Yield:	Prep time:	Serving size:
1¼ cups	10 minutes	2 tablespoons
Each serving has:		
49.2 calories	6.1 mg sodium	

1 ripe medium avocado, pitted

⅓ cup sour cream

2 TB. fresh lime juice

3 TB. water

1. Scoop avocado pulp out of rind, and purée pulp in a blender.

2. Add sour cream, lime juice, and water, and blend on high speed for 1 minute or until smooth, stopping to scrape down sides as necessary.

3. Serve immediately or chill for 30 minutes, covering surface directly with plastic wrap to prevent discoloration.

PINCH OF SAGE

This thick, creamy dressing can complement a fruit-studded green salad. Try it in the Creamy Avocado and Pink Grapefruit Toss recipe in Chapter 20.

Honey Mustard Dressing

The zest of dry mustard and the tang of yogurt are whisked together with the sweetness of honey in this classic heat-and-sweet dressing.

Yield:	Prep time:	Serving size:
⅓ cup	5 minutes	1 tablespoon
Each serving has:		
20.8 calories	6.9 mg sodium	

¼ cup fat-free plain yogurt

1 TB. honey

½ TB. fresh lemon juice

¾ to 1 tsp. dry mustard

Pinch garlic powder

Pinch onion powder

1. In a small bowl, combine yogurt, honey, lemon juice, dry mustard, garlic powder, and onion powder.

2. Whisk until well blended. Cover and chill if not serving immediately. Refrigerate any leftovers tightly covered for 3 to 5 days.

Salternative: You can adjust the honey-to-mustard ratio in this dressing to suit your taste, from sweet to spicy.

Hint-of-Lime Cucumber Dressing

Lime and garlic mingle with the garden-fresh taste of cucumber in this velvety yogurt dressing.

Yield:	Prep time:	Serving size:
1 cup	10 minutes	2 tablespoons

Each serving has:		
8.7 calories	8.5 mg sodium	

¼ medium cucumber, peeled and chopped (about ¼ cup)	¼ tsp. Salt-Shaker Substitute (recipe in Chapter 14) or other salt-free salt-substitute seasoning blend
½ cup fat-free plain yogurt	
½ tsp. fresh lime juice	
1 small clove garlic, minced	⅛ tsp. ground white pepper

1. In a blender, combine cucumber, yogurt, lime juice, garlic, Salt-Shaker Substitute, and white pepper.

2. Blend on high speed for 20 seconds or until well blended. Cover and chill if not serving immediately. Refrigerate any leftovers tightly covered for 3 to 5 days.

Salternative: If you prefer the taste of lemon juice, use it instead of the lime juice in this recipe.

Golden Garlic Dressing

This creamy, garlicky delight dresses salads with robust flavor.

Yield:	Prep time:	Chill time:	Serving size:
¾ cup	10 minutes	30 minutes	2 tablespoons
Each serving has:			
129.6 calories	8.8 mg sodium		

6 TB. extra-virgin olive oil	½ tsp. ground white pepper
6 TB. fat-free plain yogurt	4 medium cloves garlic, minced
2 tsp. fresh lemon juice	

1. In a small bowl, whisk together extra-virgin olive oil, yogurt, lemon juice, and white pepper until well combined and smooth. Whisk in garlic.

2. Cover and chill for at least 30 minutes to allow flavors to blend. Refrigerate any leftovers, tightly covered, for 3 to 5 days.

PINCH OF SAGE

Garlic lovers will enjoy this creamy dressing. You may want to reduce the amount of garlic for those not so fond of the bulb.

Raspberry Fruit Salad Dressing

Fresh red raspberries lend their summer flavor to creamy yogurt in this honey-kissed dressing.

Yield:	Prep time:	Serving size:
⅔ cup	5 minutes	2 tablespoons
Each serving has:		
35.9 calories	13 mg sodium	

½ cup fat-free plain yogurt	2 TB. honey
¼ cup red raspberries	

1. In a blender, combine yogurt, raspberries, and honey.

2. Blend on high speed for 10 seconds or until blended, stopping to scrape down the sides as necessary. Cover and chill for up to 8 hours if not serving immediately.

PINCH OF SAGE

Drizzle this dressing over a medley of your favorite fruits.

Classic Potato Salad Dressing

This creamy, mustard-tinged, tangy dressing is perfect for all your traditional picnic salads.

Yield:	Prep time:	Cook time:	Serving size:
1¾ cups	20 minutes	8 minutes	2 tablespoons
Each serving has:			
62.6 calories	14 mg sodium		

¾ cup granulated sugar

¼ cup white vinegar

¼ cup water

2 large eggs, beaten

2 TB. all-purpose flour

1 tsp. unsalted butter

½ tsp. dry mustard

½ cup fat-free plain yogurt

1. In a small saucepan, combine sugar, white vinegar, water, eggs, flour, butter, and dry mustard. Set over medium heat, and cook, stirring frequently, for 8 minutes or until mixture thickens and is smooth. Remove from heat, and cool.

2. Stir yogurt into the saucepan until mixture is well blended. Refrigerate any leftovers or salads made with this dressing tightly covered for 3 to 5 days.

PINCH OF SAGE

You can use this mayonnaise-free mixture to dress your favorite potato salad. It yields enough salad dressing for about 4 pounds potatoes. You can also try it in the Homey Macaroni Salad recipe in Chapter 20.

Creamy Herb Dressing

Oregano and basil add flavor to this smooth, yogurt-based dressing.

Yield:	Prep time:	Serving size:
1⅛ cups	10 minutes	2 tablespoons

Each serving has:		
27.4 calories	14.5 mg sodium	

1 cup fat-free, sugar-free vanilla yogurt

2 TB. red wine vinegar

1 TB. extra-virgin olive oil

¼ heaping tsp. dried basil

¼ heaping tsp. dried oregano

1 medium clove garlic, crushed

Pinch freshly ground black pepper

1. In a small bowl, combine yogurt, red wine vinegar, and extra-virgin olive oil. Whisk until blended. Whisk in basil, oregano, garlic, and pepper.

2. Serve immediately, or cover and chill, whisking again before serving. Refrigerate any leftovers tightly covered for 3 to 5 days.

Salternative: You can use fresh herbs in this salad dressing if you prefer. Substitute 1 teaspoon fresh herb for both the basil and oregano.

Soups and Stews to Savor

In This Chapter

- Sodium-sensible soup ingredients
- Dishing out bowlfuls of nutrients
- Slurping in moderation

Perhaps no other food is as homey as a soup or stew. The tempting aroma and delightful taste of a hot bowl warms your heart and your body. You're easily transported back to Mom's kitchen with all its comfort and care.

If you've stopped slurping up your favorite soups and stews because of the astonishing sodium counts, take heart. You can enjoy a cup of comfort by choosing low-sodium ingredients and sensible substitutions. Plus, if you haven't discovered cold fruit soups, you're in for a treat.

Hot or cold, a bowl of soup or a hearty stew supplies a wealth of nutrients—and now with much less sodium. So go grab your spoon!

The Pros of Soups and Stews

If soups and stews tend to be high-sodium meals, why not just eliminate them from your diet? For one, lowering your sodium intake shouldn't be about deprivation. You can enjoy many wonderfully delectable foods as long as you keep your portions in check.

Moreover, soups and stews are teeming with vitamins and minerals. None of the nutrients are poured down the drain because the cooking water is a vital part of the dish. Plus, soups and stews are packed with healthful ingredients—veggies, beans, herbs, spices, lean meats, even fruits. It's goodness you can eat with a spoon!

And with homemade soups, you can opt for low- or no-sodium ingredients. The recipes in this chapter call for fat-free, reduced-sodium canned or boxed broths. These broths are reduced in sodium by 50 percent, but they still contain a hefty serving of sodium. We chose them because they're readily available, and if you watch your serving size, these soups and stews can easily fit into your daily, low-sodium diet. Of course, if you can buy or prepare broths lower in sodium, you can substitute those in these recipes.

Tomato-based soups should be prepared with no-salt-added canned products or fresh tomatoes. The same applies to beans. Many recipes that follow call for no-salt-added canned beans for convenience. If you want to save on a bit of sodium and have time, you may prepare dried beans to substitute in any of these recipes.

PINCH OF SAGE

Don't get carried away when cooking dried beans by dumping the entire bag into the soaking water—unless you plan on using all those beans—because 1 pound dried beans (about 2 cups) yields 6 cups cooked beans.

Tri-Colored Melon Soup

Delight in the summer-sweet blend of cantaloupe, honeydew, and watermelon in this sweet cold soup.

Yield:	Prep time:	Chill time:	Serving size:
7 servings	20 minutes	1 hour	¾ cup

Each serving has:			
98.7 calories	24.7 mg sodium		

2 cups cubed cantaloupe (about ¾ small cantaloupe)

¾ cup fat-free plain yogurt

4½ TB. honey

2 cups cubed honeydew (about ½ small honeydew)

2 cups cubed seedless watermelon

1. In a blender, combine cantaloupe, ¼ cup yogurt, and 1½ tablespoons honey. Purée on high speed for 5 seconds or until blended. Transfer to a 2-cup measuring cup or small bowl.

2. In the blender, combine honeydew, ¼ cup yogurt, and 1½ tablespoons honey. Purée on high speed for 5 seconds or until blended. Transfer to a separate 2-cup measuring cup or small bowl.

3. In the blender, combine watermelon, remaining ¼ cup yogurt, and remaining 1½ tablespoons honey. Purée on high speed for 5 seconds or until blended. Transfer to a separate 2-cup measuring cup or small bowl.

4. Cover and chill separate mixtures for 1 hour.

5. In each of 7 shallow bowls or deep plates, pour ¼ cup cantaloupe mixture on 1 side and ¼ cup honeydew mixture on the other side. Pour ¼ cup watermelon mixture in the center. Using a wooden skewer or pick, swirl through the mixtures, circling clockwise. (Use a gentle hand to keep the colors from muddying.)

PINCH OF SAGE

You may need to adjust the honey according to the sweetness of the melons. Ripe fruit works well in this recipe.

Honey-Kissed Strawberry Soup

Slurp up a creamy, sweet bowl of spring-fresh strawberries.

Yield:	Prep time:	Chill time:	Serving size:
2 cups	5 minutes	1 hour	½ cup
Each serving has:			
57 calories	35.1 mg sodium		

1 cup sliced fresh strawberries	2 TB. fresh orange juice
1 cup fat-free plain yogurt	1 TB. honey

1. In a blender, combine strawberries, yogurt, orange juice, and honey. Purée on low speed for 5 seconds. Then blend on low speed for 5 to 10 more seconds, stopping to scrape down the sides if necessary.

2. Cover and chill soup for at least 1 hour before serving.

3. Stir again before serving, and garnish individual servings with a fanned fresh strawberry or a sprig of fresh mint, if desired.

Salternative: Substitute frozen unsweetened sliced strawberries, thawed and drained, when berries are out of season.

If you pick your own fresh strawberries, pluck only plump red berries from the vines. Strawberries do not ripen after they've been picked as other fruits do.

Summer Garden Cream of Tomato Soup

Spoon up fresh tomato taste in a creamy broth with a touch of thyme.

Yield:	Prep time:	Cook time:	Serving size:
5½ cups	20 minutes	35 minutes	1 cup

Each serving has:		
103.3 calories	38.2 mg sodium	

2 tsp. extra-virgin olive oil	2 tsp. cornstarch
1 medium sweet onion, thinly sliced	½ cup fat-free evaporated milk
1 bay leaf	¼ tsp. freshly ground black pepper
3 lb. (about 4 or 5 large) tomatoes, peeled, cored, seeded, and chopped	¼ tsp. dried thyme

1. In a medium-large saucepan over medium heat, heat extra-virgin olive oil. Add sweet onion and bay leaf, and cook, stirring often, for 5 minutes or until onion is softened.

2. Add tomatoes to the skillet, and bring to a simmer. Reduce heat to low, cover, and simmer for 20 minutes. Discard bay leaf.

3. Transfer tomato mixture to a blender or a food processor, and purée to desired consistency. Return to the saucepan.

4. In a small bowl, whisk together cornstarch and evaporated milk. Stir into tomato mixture. Return to a simmer over medium heat, and simmer for 5 minutes or until thickened. Stir in pepper and thyme until evenly distributed.

Don't overstir or overheat a recipe thickened with cornstarch because it may cause thinning, defeating the purpose of adding the thickening agent.

Down-Home Veggie Soup

Basil-seasoned ground beef and potatoes marry with bits of carrots, onions, celery, and tomatoes in this hot and homey soup.

Yield:	Prep time:	Cook time:	Serving size:
12 cups	10 minutes	1 hour	1 cup

Each serving has:			
128.2 calories	45.3 mg sodium		

1 lb. 85-percent-lean ground beef	1 bay leaf
2 medium yellow onions, chopped	¼ tsp. dried basil
4 cups cold water	1 TB. garlic-and-herb salt substitute seasoning blend
10 baby carrots, cut on the diagonal	6 large tomatoes, peeled, cored, and chopped
2 ribs celery, thinly sliced	
2 medium potatoes, peeled and chopped	

1. In a medium nonstick skillet over medium heat, brown ground beef. With a slotted spoon, transfer ground beef to a paper towel–lined plate to drain. Drain the skillet but do not dry.

2. Add onions to the skillet, reduce heat to medium-low, and sauté for 5 minutes or until just turning golden.

3. In a large soup pot, combine onions, cold water, carrots, celery, potatoes, bay leaf, basil, and garlic-and-herb salt substitute seasoning blend. Bring to a boil. Reduce heat as needed to maintain a simmer, cover, and simmer for 30 minutes.

4. Stir in ground beef and tomatoes, and return to a boil. Reduce heat as needed to maintain a simmer, cover, and simmer for 10 minutes or until vegetables are tender. Discard bay leaf before serving.

PINCH OF SAGE

To easily peel tomatoes, place them in boiling water for 10 to 15 seconds. Remove with tongs. When cool enough to handle, peel with the tip of a sharp knife and your fingers.

Slow-Simmered Minestrone

The rich, well-seasoned beef-and-tomato broth provides a rich base for veggies, beans, and pasta.

Yield:	Prep time:	Cook time:	Serving size:
9 cups	10 minutes	4 or 5 hours	1 cup

Each serving has:	
116.4 calories	63 mg sodium

1 small yellow onion, diced

6 large baby carrots, halved and sliced

2 ribs celery, diced

1 cup chopped green cabbage

2 medium cloves garlic, minced

1 tsp. dried basil

1 tsp. dried marjoram

½ tsp. dried oregano

¼ tsp. freshly ground black pepper

2 (14.5-oz.) cans light-sodium, fat-free beef broth

1 (15-oz.) can no-salt-added tomato sauce

1 (14.5-oz.) can no-salt-added diced tomatoes

1 (15-oz.) can no-salt-added Great Northern beans, drained

¼ cup *pastina*

1. In a 5-quart slow cooker, combine onion, carrots, celery, cabbage, garlic, basil, marjoram, oregano, pepper, beef broth, tomato sauce, diced tomatoes, and Great Northern beans. Cover and cook on high for 4 or 5 hours or on low heat for 8 to 10 hours.

2. Stir in pastina during the last 15 to 30 minutes of cooking time. Cover and cook until pastina is tender.

Salternative: Save on a bit of sodium by substituting 2 cups cooked Great Northern beans.

DEFINITION

Pastina is Italian for "little dough" and is simply a very small pasta. You can use any tiny pasta shape, such as acini de pepe or alphabets.

Farmhouse Oven Beef Stew

A thick, seasoned broth carries tender beef with potatoes and carrots.

Yield:	Prep time:	Cook time:	Serving size:
6 cups	10 minutes	2 hours, 40 minutes	1 cup

Each serving has:	
374 calories	134.8 mg sodium

1½ TB. extra-light olive oil

¼ cup all-purpose flour

¾ tsp. freshly ground black pepper

¼ tsp. garlic powder

1½ lb. lean stew beef cubes

2 medium yellow onions, chopped

3 ribs celery, sliced

12 large baby carrots, sliced

2 cups low-sodium vegetable juice

1½ cups water

½ cup quick-cooking tapioca

½ tsp. dried basil

1 TB. granulated sugar

1 bay leaf

3 medium all-purpose potatoes, peeled and chopped

1. Preheat the oven to 325°F. Spray a deep, 3-quart casserole dish with nonstick cooking spray.

2. In a large nonstick skillet over medium heat, heat extra-light olive oil.

3. In a shallow dish, stir together flour, ¼ teaspoon pepper, and garlic powder. Dredge beef cubes in seasoned flour, shaking off excess. Add beef to the skillet, and brown on all sides.

4. Transfer beef to the prepared casserole dish. Top with onions, celery, and carrots.

5. In a medium bowl, combine vegetable juice, 1 cup water, tapioca, basil, remaining ½ teaspoon pepper, sugar, and bay leaf. Stir and pour over beef mixture. Cover and bake for 2 hours.

6. Add potatoes and remaining ½ cup water to the casserole dish, and stir. Cover and bake for 30 to 40 minutes or until potatoes are tender.

Salternative: This stew is thick. If you prefer a thinner stew, reduce the amount of tapioca as desired.

PINCH OF SAGE

Add small whole fresh mushrooms or sliced fresh mushrooms with the potatoes if you like. Fresh mushrooms will add just a few milligrams of sodium: 4 milligrams for 1 cup whole or 1½ milligrams for ½ cup slices.

Split-Pea Soup with Mini Meatballs

The classic pea flavor is accompanied by sweet, rosemary-flavored turkey meatballs.

Yield:	Prep time:	Cook time:	Serving size:
6 servings	10 minutes	1 hour, 50 minutes	1 cup soup with about 8 meatballs

Each serving has:	
232.5 calories	153.9 mg sodium

1 TB. extra-light olive oil

1 medium yellow onion, finely chopped (about 1 cup)

2 ribs celery, finely chopped

1 medium clove garlic, minced

1½ tsp. dried crushed rosemary

1 (48-oz.) can *light-sodium* fat-free chicken broth (6 cups)

1¼ cups dried green split peas, sorted and rinsed

½ lb. ground turkey

¼ tsp. freshly ground black pepper

1. In a large soup pot over medium heat, heat extra-light olive oil. Add onion, celery, garlic, and 1 teaspoon rosemary, and sauté for 5 minutes or until softened, stirring frequently.

2. Pour in chicken broth, add split peas, and stir. Increase heat to high, and bring to a boil. Reduce heat as needed to maintain a simmer, cover, and simmer for 1½ hours or until split peas are tender. Remove from heat, and let cool.

3. Meanwhile, in a large bowl, combine ground turkey, pepper, and remaining ½ teaspoon rosemary until seasonings are evenly distributed. Form into about 4 dozen tiny ½-inch meatballs.

4. In a large nonstick skillet over medium heat, brown meatballs on all sides for 7 to 10 minutes or until cooked through and no pink remains. Using a slotted spoon, remove meatballs to a paper towel–lined plate to drain.

5. Ladle about $\frac{1}{2}$ soup or more into a blender or food processor. Purée on high speed for 15 seconds or until smooth. Return to the pot, add meatballs, and stir. Increase heat to medium-high, and bring to a slow simmer to heat through.

> **DEFINITION**
>
> **Light sodium** refers to a product that has at least 50 percent less sodium than the regular product. Check the nutrition label for actual sodium amounts. (Labels are now moving away from this term toward the more general use of "reduced sodium," so be certain to check sodium contents.)

Roasted Poblano Pepper and Chicken Stew

The smoky heat of hot *poblano peppers* infuses this stew full of juicy chicken and chunks of sweet potatoes.

Yield:	Prep time:	Cook time:	Serving size:
4 cups	25 minutes	40 minutes	1 cup
Each serving has:			
225.5 calories	195.7 mg sodium		

3 medium poblano peppers

1 tsp. extra-virgin olive oil

1 lb. chicken breast, cut into 2-in. cubes

1 cup diced yellow onions

1 tsp. Salt-Shaker Substitute (recipe in Chapter 14) or other salt-free salt substitute seasoning blend

1 medium clove garlic, minced

1 cup reduced-sodium, fat-free chicken broth

1 medium sweet potato, coarsely chopped

1 TB. chopped fresh cilantro

$\frac{1}{8}$ tsp. freshly ground black pepper

1 TB. all-purpose flour

2 TB. cold water

1. Preheat the broiler to high.

2. Wash whole poblano peppers, and arrange on a small baking sheet. Broil on the top oven rack for 4 minutes or until exposed skin is well charred. Remove from the oven, and using tongs, turn peppers over. Broil for 4 more minutes or until well charred. Immediately place peppers in a small brown paper bag, close tightly, and allow peppers to steam for 15 minutes.

3. Remove peppers from the bag and, working over a small bowl, peel skins from peppers with your fingers. Cut peppers lengthwise, and cut away and discard the tops with the stems. Scrape out and discard seeds. Chop roasted peppers, and set aside.

4. Heat a large saucepan over medium heat. When hot, add extra-virgin olive oil, and heat for 1 minute. Add chicken, onions, and Salt-Shaker Substitute, and cook for 5 minutes, stirring frequently to brown chicken on all sides. Stir in garlic, and cook for 1 more minute.

5. Slowly stir in chicken broth. Add sweet potato and poblano peppers, and stir. Bring to a boil, cover, and reduce heat as needed to maintain a simmer. Simmer for 25 minutes or until sweet potatoes are tender.

6. Add cilantro and pepper, and stir.

7. In a small container with a lid, combine flour and cold water. Cover and shake until blended. Add to stew, and stir to thicken slightly. Serve stew over cooked brown rice or other grain, as desired.

Salternative: For a less-spicy stew, substitute one or more green or red bell peppers for the poblano peppers.

DEFINITION

Poblano peppers are dark green, tapered peppers best known perhaps for their use in chiles rellenos recipes. The poblano pepper isn't as hot as a jalpeño pepper, but it does have a bit of a kick.

One-Pot Cajun Shrimp Stew

A rich *roux* deepens the taste of the gravy in which succulent shrimp swim.

Yield:	Prep time:	Cook time:	Serving size:
4 cups	5 minutes	55 minutes	1 cup

Each serving has:		
240.1 calories	198.8 mg sodium	

2 TB. trans-fat-free soft vegetable shortening	3 medium cloves garlic, minced
3 TB. all-purpose flour	2 TB. no-salt-added tomato sauce
1 large green bell pepper, ribs and seeds removed, and chopped	1 cup water
1 medium yellow onion, chopped	1 lb. medium shrimp (about 46), peeled and deveined, cooked or uncooked
1 small rib celery, diced	

1. In a large saucepan over medium heat, melt vegetable shortening. Whisk in flour, and cook, whisking, for 5 minutes or until roux is deep golden brown.

2. Reduce heat to low, and add green bell pepper, onion, celery, and garlic. Cover and cook for 10 minutes.

3. Add tomato sauce and water to the saucepan. Cover and simmer for 30 minutes.

4. Stir shrimp into the saucepan. Cover and gently simmer for 10 minutes. Remove from heat, and serve stew over cooked long-grain brown rice, if desired.

DEFINITION

Roux is a French word for a fat-and-flour mixture. This recipe calls for a medium roux, which should be about the color of peanut butter. Be sure to whisk your roux *constantly*—that means you can't answer the phone, get the door, or chop the vegetables. You'll need to do that before you start cooking.

Two-Bean Turkey Chili

Pintos and black beans join ground turkey in a traditional spiced tomato base.

Yield:	Prep time:	Cook time:	Serving size:
7 cups	5 minutes	1 hour, 40 minutes	1 cup

Each serving has:			
210.6 calories	226 mg sodium		

¾ lb. ground turkey

2 small yellow onions, chopped

1 medium green bell pepper, ribs and seeds removed, and chopped

1 (14.5-oz.) can no-salt-added diced tomatoes, with juice

1 (15-oz.) can no-salt-added tomato sauce

1 (15-oz.) can no-salt-added pinto beans, rinsed and drained

1 (15-oz.) can no-salt-added black beans, rinsed and drained

2½ tsp. Firehouse Chili Powder (recipe in Chapter 14) or other salt-free chili powder

1½ tsp. Salt-Shaker Substitute (recipe in Chapter 14) or other salt-free salt substitute seasoning blend

¼ tsp. paprika

¼ tsp. ground ginger

1. In a large saucepan over medium heat, brown ground turkey with onions and green bell pepper for 7 minutes or until meat is browned and onions are translucent. Drain well.

2. Add diced tomatoes, tomato sauce, pinto beans, and black beans, and stir. Add Firehouse Chili Powder, Salt-Shaker Substitute, paprika, and ginger, and stir. Bring to a boil. Reduce heat as needed to maintain a simmer, cover, and simmer for 1½ hours.

PINCH OF SAGE

You can substitute any two of your favorite beans in this recipe—kidney beans, Great Northern beans, pink beans, and so on. Just keep them low in sodium.

French Onion Soup

Packed with slow-sautéed onions, this rich, seasoned beef broth is topped with seasoned bread cubes and Swiss cheese.

Yield:	Prep time:	Cook time:	Serving size:
2 servings	5 minutes	43 minutes	1 cup soup plus toppings

Each serving has:	
367.3 calories	292.2 mg sodium

1 TB. extra-virgin olive oil

3 cups thinly sliced and halved yellow onions

2½ cups unsalted beef stock

1 bay leaf

1 small clove garlic, peeled, trimmed, and halved lengthwise

1 TB. all-purpose flour

1½ tsp. Salt-Shaker Substitute (recipe in Chapter 14) or other salt-free salt substitute seasoning blend

¼ tsp. freshly ground black pepper

½ cup Garlic-Pepper Croutons (recipe in Chapter 6)

½ cup coarsely shredded low-sodium Swiss cheese

1. Heat a very large skillet over medium-low heat. When hot, add extra-virgin olive oil, and heat for 1 minute. Add onions, stir to coat, and cook for 30 minutes or until translucent and tender, stirring frequently to avoid browning.

2. Meanwhile, in a large saucepan over medium heat, combine beef stock, bay leaf, and garlic. Bring to a simmer, and simmer while onions cook.

3. Stir flour into onions, and cook for 1 minute.

4. Meanwhile, remove bay leaf and garlic from beef stock. Stir in Salt-Shaker Substitute and pepper. Add onion mixture, stirring. Cook for 10 minutes, returning to a simmer and reducing heat as needed to maintain a simmer.

5. Preheat the broiler to high.

6. Spoon 1 cup soup into each of 2 small oven-proof serving bowls. Top each with ¼ cup Garlic-Pepper Croutons, and sprinkle ¼ cup Swiss cheese on top. Broil 4 inches from the heat source for 1 or 2 minutes or until cheese is bubbly, watching carefully. Serve immediately.

SALT PITFALL

Swiss cheese may not be labeled low-sodium because the cheese may be naturally low in sodium—about 30 milligrams per 1-ounce serving. Watch the nutrition data information, though, because some versions are just as high in sodium as other cheeses.

Black Bean and Brown Rice Soup

Lightly seasoned chicken broth serves up healthful black beans and brown rice.

Yield:	Prep time:	Cook time:	Serving size:
6 cups	5 minutes	50 minutes	1 cup

Each serving has:			
178.6 calories	303.1 mg sodium		

2 tsp. extra-virgin olive oil	2 cups cooked, drained black beans
1 cup finely chopped yellow onions	1 TB. red wine vinegar
2 medium cloves garlic, minced	½ tsp. Salt-Shaker Substitute (recipe in Chapter 14) or other salt-free salt substitute seasoning blend
½ tsp. ground cumin	
½ tsp. dried oregano	
⅛ tsp. crushed red pepper flakes	2 cups cooked brown rice
4 cups reduced-sodium, fat-free chicken broth	

1. Heat a large saucepan over medium heat. When hot, add extra-virgin olive oil, and heat for 1 minute. Add onions and cook, stirring frequently, for 3 minutes or until golden.

2. Add garlic, cumin, oregano, and crushed red pepper flakes. Cook, stirring, for 1 minute.

3. Slowly add chicken broth, and stir in black beans. Increase heat to high, and bring to a boil. Reduce heat to low, cover, and simmer for 30 minutes.

4. Remove 1 cup black bean mixture to a food processor and blend on high speed for 15 seconds or until smooth. Return to the saucepan.

5. Add red wine vinegar, Salt-Shaker Substitute, and brown rice. Cover, reduce heat to low, and simmer for 10 minutes or until heated through.

Sensational Sandwiches

In This Chapter

- Satisfying low-sodium sandwiches
- Finding low-sodium breads
- Sodium-responsible condiments and other fixings
- Open up to open-face sandwiches

Nothing says lunch like a sandwich. From the humble PB&J to a gourmet roasted egg-plant and fresh mozzarella with roasted red pepper relish on focaccia, a good sandwich hits the spot at midday.

For people on a sodium-restricted diet, eating a simple sandwich can become a complicated endeavor. Regular breads are high in sodium. Deli lunch meats contain incredibly high amounts of sodium. And of course, we must have condiments—pickles, relish, mustard, ketchup, mayonnaise, salsa, barbecue sauce, hot pepper sauce, steak sauce, and salad dressings make building a sandwich a sodium landmine field. Should we even mention cheese?

Fortunately, you can find ingredients that will fit your low-sodium meal plan. With a little ingenuity, you can sink your teeth into a satisfying lunchtime sandwich without a care. Is that the lunch bell ringing?

It's All About the Bread

A sandwich isn't really a sandwich without the bread, right? (Well, we do have a tasty recipe that eliminates the bread: Turkey and Swiss in a Green Blanket.) But you're at a loss as to how to find suitable breads for your needs.

An online search can give you a few sources for low-sodium and even salt-free breads. Some companies will ship the breads to your home. So if you can afford slightly higher prices and shipping charges, your problem is solved.

But also check out your own neighborhood for lo-so bread. You may be pleasantly surprised. Some supermarkets carry commercially made low-sodium breads, or their in-store bakeries may offer low-sodium options. You won't know until you ask. Smaller grocers often offer selections that differ from the large supermarket conglomerates. They may also be able to order low-sodium breads in small quantities from their distributors—again, ask. Local bakeries are another good place to poke around. You might have to special order low-sodium loaves, rolls, or buns, but that's easy enough.

If you're simply unable to get your hands on low-sodium breads, you'll have to work with what's available. Perhaps the quickest solution is to make an open-faced sandwich. Using a single slice of bread automatically cuts the amount of sodium from the bread in a sandwich in half. Plus, some regularly available sandwich holders are okay in terms of sodium content. You can usually incorporate a regular corn taco shell, half an English muffin, or half a regular bun into your diet without spoiling your sodium count.

> **PINCH OF SAGE**
>
> Another option for a low-sodium sandwich wrap is to use a crepe from the Lemon Raspberry Crepes recipe in Chapter 4. See the recipe for Sautéed Spinach and Mushroom Crepes, later in this chapter, as well.

Sandwich Snafus Avoided

With the high sodium in condiments, meats, and cheeses, what's left to put on your sandwich? Many regular condiments are available in no-salt-added or low-sodium versions. If you prefer, prepare your own sodium-wise condiments from the recipes offered in Chapter 12.

If you'd like a classic deli meat sandwich, you'll have to be alert. Typical deli meats contain astronomical amounts of sodium. Some manufacturers, such as Boar's Head, Sara Lee, and Dietz & Watson, produce lower-sodium turkey, ham, or roast beef products. Ask if your deli department has lower-sodium options.

And if you top your sandwich with cheese, make it a low-sodium variety.

Southwestern Portobello and Black Bean Burgers

Crisp on the outside and tender on the inside, these veggie burgers are flavored with fresh cilantro.

Yield:	Prep time:	Cook time:	Serving size:
4 burgers	5 minutes	18 minutes	1 burger

Each serving has:		
320.2 calories	5.7 mg sodium	

2 tsp. extra-virgin olive oil

1/4 cup diced yellow onions

2 medium cloves garlic, minced

2 cups finely chopped baby portobello or crimini mushrooms

1/2 tsp. ground cumin

1 cup cooked black beans, drained

1/3 cup chopped fresh cilantro

1 3/4 cups sodium-free sprouted-grain breadcrumbs

2 tsp. Salt-Shaker Substitute (recipe in Chapter 14) or other salt-free salt substitute seasoning blend

1/2 tsp. freshly ground black pepper

4 Whole-Wheat Sandwich Flats (recipe in Chapter 19), split, or other low-sodium sandwich buns

1. Preheat a double-sided indoor grill.

2. Heat a large skillet over medium heat. When hot, add extra-virgin olive oil. Add onions, and cook, stirring frequently, for 5 minutes or until golden brown.

3. Add garlic and cook, stirring, for 1 minute. Add mushrooms and cumin. Cook, stirring occasionally, for 5 minutes or until mushrooms release their liquid.

4. In a food processor, combine mushroom mixture, black beans, and cilantro. Process on high speed for 30 seconds or until mixed, stopping to scrape down the sides as necessary.

5. In a large bowl, combine black bean mixture, breadcrumbs, Salt-Shaker Substitute, and pepper, and stir until blended. Shape into 4 (4-inch) patties.

6. Cook patties for 5 to 7 minutes or until outsides are crisp and patties are heated through. Serve on Whole-Wheat Sandwich Flats with low-sodium burger toppings as desired.

Salternative: If you prefer to prepare these burgers in the broiler, place patties on the rack of a broiler pan coated with nonstick cooking spray and broil on high 6 inches from the heat source for 10 minutes or until crisped, turning burgers halfway through cooking time.

PINCH OF SAGE

To prepare breadcrumbs, tear bread slices into rough pieces and place in a food processor. Process until fine, even crumbs form. Measure as needed.

Rosemary Turkey Burgers

These hearty, lean burgers are moist and seasoned with a hint of rosemary.

Yield:	Prep time:	Cook time:	Serving size:
5 burgers	5 minutes	10 minutes	1 burger

Each serving has:			
298.2 calories	58.5 mg sodium		

1¼ lb. 99-percent fat-free extra-lean ground turkey breast

⅓ cup natural raw wheat germ

2 TB. fat-free milk

1 large egg, at room temperature

½ TB. Salt-Shaker Substitute (recipe in Chapter 14) or other salt-free salt substitute seasoning blend

¼ tsp. dried crushed rosemary

5 Whole-Wheat Sandwich Flats (recipe in Chapter 19), split, or other low-sodium sandwich buns

1. Preheat the broiler to high. Coat the rack of a broiler pan with nonstick cooking spray.

2. In a medium bowl, combine ground turkey breast, wheat germ, milk, egg, Salt-Shaker Substitute, and rosemary. Using your hands, mix until evenly blended, and divide into 5 equal portions. Shape each portion into a ½-inch-thick patty, and place on the rack of the broiler pan.

3. Broil 4 to 6 inches from the heat source for 10 minutes, turning halfway through cooking time, or until done (165°F on a food thermometer). Serve on Whole-Wheat Sandwich Flats. Garnish with sodium-free or low-sodium condiments and sliced vegetables as desired.

PINCH OF SAGE

Wheat germ makes a good sodium-free substitute for breadcrumbs in many recipes. Look for it in the cereal aisle or health food section of your supermarket.

Sautéed Spinach and Mushrooms Crepes

A thin, tender wrap encloses spicy hummus and meaty portobello mushrooms with wilted spinach.

Yield:	Prep time:	Cook time:	Serving size:
6 crepes	15 minutes	16 minutes	2 crepes

Each serving has:			
261.8 calories	60.2 mg sodium		

1 large egg, at room temperature

$\frac{1}{4}$ cup fat-free milk

$\frac{1}{4}$ cup water

$\frac{1}{2}$ cup all-purpose flour

1 TB. unsalted butter, melted

1 TB. extra-virgin olive oil

6 ($\frac{1}{2}$-in.-thick) slices portobello mushroom caps

2 cups packed baby spinach leaves

$\frac{1}{2}$ tsp. garlic powder

$\frac{1}{2}$ tsp. onion powder

6 TB. Zippy Jalapeño Hummus (recipe in Chapter 10)

1. In a medium bowl, blend together egg, milk, and water. Stir in flour and butter. Let batter stand for 20 minutes.

2. Meanwhile, heat a large nonstick skillet over medium heat. When hot, add extra-virgin olive oil, and heat for 30 seconds. Stir in mushrooms, and cook, stirring occasionally, for 7 minutes or until mushrooms release their liquid.

3. Stir in spinach, garlic powder, and onion powder, and cook, stirring often, for 2 minutes or until spinach is wilted. Set aside, keeping warm.

4. Heat a medium nonstick skillet over medium heat. Coat the skillet with nonstick cooking spray. Pour about 3 tablespoons batter into the skillet for each crepe, tilting the skillet to spread batter to a 6-inch diameter. Cook for 30 seconds or until edges are dry and underside is golden. Turn and cook for 20 to 30 more seconds or until underside is golden. Remove crepe to a sheet of waxed paper or a plate, and repeat with remaining batter.

5. Spread 1 tablespoon Zippy Jalapeño Hummus over each crepe, and top with 1 mushroom slice and spinach. Fold over sides of crepes to serve.

PINCH OF SAGE

Look for packaged thick-sliced portobello mushroom caps in your grocer's produce section to make this sandwich even simpler to prepare.

Pulled Pork and Slaw Sandwich

This filling sandwich is meaty and spicy with a touch of crunch.

Yield:	Prep time:	Serving size:
1 sandwich	2 minutes	½ sandwich
Each serving has:		
309.1 calories	94.2 mg sodium	

1 cup pulled Slow Cooker Saucy Pork Shoulder Roast (recipe in Chapter 17)

½ cup Zesty Vinaigrette Coleslaw (recipe in Chapter 20)

2 slices sodium-free sprouted-grain bread or other sodium-free bread

1. Pile pulled Slow Cooker Saucy Pork Shoulder Roast and Zesty Vinaigrette Coleslaw on 1 slice sprouted-grain bread and top with remaining bread slice.

2. Cut in half diagonally to serve.

PINCH OF SAGE

To pull pork, use two forks or your fingers to shred pork slices and toss with liquid reduction from the Slow Cooker Saucy Pork Shoulder Roast recipe.

Broiled Cheese-Capped Salad Sandwiches

A toasted bread slice serves as the foundation for fresh veggies topped with melty cheddar cheese.

Yield:	Prep time:	Cook time:	Serving size:
6 sandwiches	15 minutes	3 minutes	1 sandwich

Each serving has:			
226.9 calories	156.7 mg sodium		

6 slices salt-free whole-wheat bread	1 medium red bell pepper, ribs and seeds removed, and chopped
2 medium tomatoes, cored and chopped	2 tsp. extra-virgin olive oil
1 large yellow onion, chopped	6 (1-oz.) slices low-sodium cheddar cheese
1 medium green bell pepper, ribs and seeds removed, and chopped	

1. Preheat the broiler to high.

2. Place bread slices on a baking sheet. Broil 4 to 6 inches from heat for 2 minutes or until bread is lightly toasted, watching carefully to avoid burning. Turn bread slices over.

3. Meanwhile, in a large bowl, combine tomatoes, onion, green bell pepper, and red bell pepper.

4. Divide vegetable mixture evenly among toasted bread slices. Lightly drizzle extra-virgin olive oil over vegetables, and top each sandwich with 1 slice cheddar cheese. Broil for 1 or 2 more minutes or until cheese is melted.

PINCH OF SAGE

If you have trouble finding salt-free whole-wheat bread, substitute regular bread with the lowest sodium content possible. The open-face nature of this sandwich should help you stay within your sodium intake goals, even with a slice of regular bread.

Quick and Easy Beefy Tacos

Sink your teeth into this traditional beef taco with lo-so accompaniments.

Yield:	Prep time:	Cook time:	Serving size:
4 tacos	5 minutes	7 minutes	1 taco

Each serving has:	
250.7 calories	174.5 mg sodium

½ lb. 85-percent-lean ground beef

¾ tsp. Taco Seasoning Mix (recipe in Chapter 14)

4 sodium-free yellow corn taco shells

½ cup finely shredded low-sodium cheddar cheese

1 cup shredded lettuce

½ cup finely diced tomatoes

1. In a small nonstick skillet over medium heat, brown ground beef with Taco Seasoning Mix. Stir, breaking up meat, until cooked through and no pink remains. Using a slotted spoon, remove beef to a paper towel–lined plate.

2. Warm taco shells according to package directions. Fill each with ¼ ground beef, 2 tablespoons cheddar cheese, ¼ cup lettuce, and 2 tablespoons tomatoes.

PINCH OF SAGE

If you have a hard time finding sodium-free taco shells, use regular taco shells. They're fairly low in sodium and more readily available.

Open-Face Cheese Steak Sandwiches

Here, seasoned thin steak is smothered in sautéed onions and cheddar sauce.

Yield:	Prep time:	Cook time:	Serving size:
2 sandwiches	8 minutes	12 minutes	1 sandwich

Each serving has:			
555.3 calories	200.3 mg sodium		

3 tsp. extra-light olive oil

1 small yellow onion, halved and sliced

$\frac{1}{2}$ lb. thin sandwich steak, trimmed of all visible fat

$\frac{1}{4}$ tsp. freshly ground black pepper

$\frac{1}{4}$ tsp. garlic powder

$\frac{1}{4}$ tsp. onion powder

1 tsp. cornstarch

$\frac{1}{4}$ cup fat-free milk

$\frac{1}{4}$ cup finely shredded low-sodium cheddar cheese

1 whole-wheat hot dog bun, split and toasted

1. In a small skillet over medium heat, heat 1 teaspoon extra-light olive oil. Add onion, and sauté for 5 minutes or until tender and golden. Remove from heat.

2. In a large, nonstick skillet over medium heat, heat remaining 2 teaspoons extra-light olive oil.

3. Cut steak into 1-inch strips, and season with pepper, garlic powder, and onion powder. Add steak to the large skillet, and cook for $1\frac{1}{2}$ minutes. Turn and cook the other side for 1 more minute or until done (160°F on a food thermometer for medium). Drain on a paper towel–lined plate.

4. In a small saucepan, whisk cornstarch into milk until blended. Heat over medium heat just until bubbles form around the edge of the pan. Reduce heat to low, and slowly whisk in cheddar cheese until melted and smooth. Remove from heat.

5. To assemble, pile steak onto each bun half. Top with onions, and pour cheese sauce over all.

Salternative: You can substitute thinly sliced beef sirloin or roast beef if you can't find thin sandwich steak. Cook it to 160°F to 170°F.

PINCH OF SAGE

If you purchase or prepare low-sodium sandwich buns—or better yet salt-free buns—feel free to enjoy this sandwich on a whole bun. Just be sure it falls within your daily dietary needs.

Turkey and Pinto Bean Soft Tacos

Taco-spiced ground turkey and pinto beans team up with favorite toppings in these surprising tacos.

Yield:	Prep time:	Cook time:	Serving size:
4 tacos	10 minutes	10 minutes	1 taco

Each serving has:	
631 calories	267.3 mg sodium

1 lb. ground turkey or 99-percent fat-free ground turkey breast

1½ tsp. Taco Seasoning Mix (recipe in Chapter 14)

½ cup finely diced yellow onions

1 (15-oz.) can no-salt-added pinto beans, rinsed and drained

4 Fresh Tortillas (recipe in Chapter 19) or other low-sodium tortillas, warmed

½ cup finely shredded low-sodium cheddar cheese

½ cup finely diced tomatoes

½ cup fat-free sour cream

1. In a large nonstick skillet over medium heat, brown ground turkey with Taco Seasoning Mix and onions. Cook for 7 or 8 minutes or until browned and no pink remains, stirring to break up meat.

2. Stir in pinto beans, and cook for 1 minute or until heated through. Using a slotted spoon, remove turkey mixture to a paper towel–lined plate.

3. Spoon turkey mixture down center of warmed Fresh Tortillas. Sprinkle on cheddar cheese and tomatoes, and spoon on sour cream. Serve, folding over, burrito-style.

PINCH OF SAGE

You can quickly warm each tortilla in the microwave on 50 percent power for 15 to 30 seconds. Preparing the tacos while the tortillas are warm and malleable helps keep them from cracking while you're folding them.

Classic Tomato Sandwich

Lightly peppered garden-fresh tomatoes sit atop toasted, buttered bread.

Yield:	Prep time:	Cook time:	Serving size:
1 sandwich	5 minutes	2 minutes	1 sandwich
Each serving has:			
224 calories	301 mg sodium		

2 slices salt-free whole-wheat bread

1½ tsp. unsalted butter

1 medium tomato, cored and thickly sliced

Pinch ground black pepper

1. Toast bread slices as desired.

2. Spread ¾ teaspoon butter on each slice.

3. Place tomato slices on buttered side of 1 bread slice. Season with pepper. Close sandwich, placing remaining bread slice butter-side down. Cut on the diagonal, if desired.

PINCH OF SAGE

If you prefer, you may omit the black pepper. Or if you like your tomato sandwiches well seasoned, sprinkle on a salt-free salt substitute seasoning blend.

Chunky Tuna Salad Pita Pockets

Creamy, tangy tuna and cheddar pair up in wheaty pita pockets.

Yield:	Prep time:	Cook time:	Serving size:
2 pita pockets	10 minutes	3 minutes	1 pita pocket
Each serving has:			
288 calories	307.4 mg sodium		

1 TB. fresh lemon juice

2 medium green onions, trimmed and sliced

1 (6-oz.) can very low-sodium albacore tuna packed in water, drained and coarsely flaked

¼ cup fat-free plain yogurt

3 TB. finely shredded low-sodium cheddar cheese

2 no-salt-added whole-wheat pita pockets

2 medium green-leaf lettuce leaves

4 thin slices tomato

1. In a small, nonstick skillet over medium heat, heat lemon juice just until hot. Add green onions, and cook for 1 or 2 minutes or until softened.

2. Add tuna, and cook for 1 or 2 minutes or until heated through. Remove from heat.

3. Stir in yogurt, evenly coating tuna. Stir in cheddar cheese.

4. Line each pita pocket with 1 lettuce leaf, spoon in tuna salad, and add 2 tomato slices to each pita pocket.

SALT PITFALL

Read those nutrition labels carefully! The tuna used in this recipe has 35 milligrams sodium per serving, but the can lists the number of servings as 2½. The cheddar cheese that's labeled "low sodium" has just 5 milligrams sodium per ounce.

Salmon Swiss Melts with Avocado

Here, creamy salmon is spread on a whole-grain English muffin and topped with avocado slices and bubbly Swiss cheese.

Yield:	Prep time:	Cook time:	Serving size:
2 melts	20 minutes	1 minute	1 English muffin half
Each serving has:			
396 calories	317.5 mg sodium		

1 (7.5-oz.) can no-salt-added pink
   salmon, drained

2 TB. finely diced green bell pepper

1/3 cup fat-free plain yogurt

1 whole-grain English muffin, split
   and toasted

1 lemon wedge

2 lengthwise slices avocado, halved

2 (1-oz.) slices low-sodium Swiss
   cheese

1. Preheat the broiler to high.

2. Flake salmon flesh into a medium bowl, discarding any skin and bones. Stir in bell pepper and yogurt until evenly distributed. Spoon salmon mixture onto English muffin halves.

3. Rub lemon wedge over avocado slices to prevent discoloration. Place 2 avocado slice halves on each English muffin half, and top with Swiss cheese slices.

4. Place sandwiches on a baking sheet, and broil 4 to 6 inches from the heat source for 1 or 2 minutes or until cheese is bubbly and melted.

 PINCH OF SAGE

If you want a sandwich even lower in sodium, substitute the English muffin with 2 slices salt-free whole-wheat bread. Toast the bread, and proceed as directed.

Honey-Barbecue Chicken Breast on Toast

Sweet and spicy thin-sliced chicken sits atop toasted whole-wheat bread.

Yield:	Prep time:	Cook time:	Serving size:
1 sandwich	5 minutes	4 minutes	1 sandwich

Each serving has:	
337.5 calories	335.8 mg sodium

1½ TB. honey

1 tsp. paprika

½ tsp. dry mustard

¼ tsp. ground cayenne

1 (2.5-oz.) thin-sliced boneless, skinless chicken breast, rinsed and patted dry with paper towels

2 slices salt-free whole-wheat bread, toasted

1 medium green-leaf lettuce leaf

2 thin slices tomato

1 (⅛- to ¼-in.-thick) slice sweet onion, separated into rings

1. In a small bowl, combine honey, paprika, dry mustard, and cayenne. Stir to blend.

2. Heat a small nonstick skillet over medium heat, then spray with nonstick cooking spray. Add chicken, and cook for 1 or 2 minutes or until browned on underside. Turn and cook for 1 more minute or until done (170°F on a food thermometer).

3. Spoon honey mixture over chicken, and cook for 30 to 60 seconds, turning chicken to coat. Remove from heat.

4. Line 1 slice of toast with lettuce. Add tomato slices and onion rings, and place chicken with sauce over top. Close sandwich with remaining slice of toast. Cut sandwich in half, and serve immediately.

PINCH OF SAGE

If you can't find salt-free bread, you can serve this recipe as an open-face sandwich, using a single slice of a whole-grain bread that has the lowest sodium content you can find. Or opt for sodium-free sprouted grain bread slices.

Turkey and Swiss in a Green Blanket

Turkey and Swiss cheese marry with sautéed peppers and onions wrapped in crisp lettuce.

Yield:	Prep time:	Cook time:	Serving size:
1 sandwich	5 minutes	6 minutes	1 sandwich

Each serving has:	
259.8 calories	371.9 mg sodium

1 tsp. extra-virgin olive oil

¼ medium red bell pepper, ribs and seeds removed, and thinly sliced

1 (¼-in.-thick) slice sweet onion, separated into rings

2 large leaves red-leaf lettuce

2 oz. skinless, 47-percent-lower-sodium deli turkey breast, chopped or sliced

2 or 3 tsp. Home-Style Mustard (recipe in Chapter 12)

1 (1-oz.) slice low-sodium Swiss cheese

1. In a small skillet over medium heat, heat extra-virgin olive oil. Add red bell pepper and sweet onion, and cook, stirring frequently, for 5 minutes or until softened.

2. Wash and dry lettuce. Place on a plate, overlapping edges of leaves. Layer turkey over top, leaving a small margin on all sides. Spread on Home-Style Mustard, and top with Swiss cheese. Scatter red bell pepper mixture over all.

3. Just before eating, wrap lettuce around filling, burrito-style.

PINCH OF SAGE

Swiss cheese is naturally lower in sodium than other traditional cheeses, but you can save on some sodium if you try this sandwich without cheese.

Big Beefy Burgers

Serve these seasoned beef hamburgers on whole-wheat rolls with all your favorite lo-so toppings.

Yield:	Prep time:	Cook time:	Serving size:
4 burgers	10 minutes	10 minutes	1 burger

Each serving has:			
458.2 calories	387.5 mg sodium		

1 lb. 85-percent-lean ground beef

½ small yellow onion, minced

¼ cup unsalted matzo meal

¼ cup no-salt-added tomato sauce

1½ tsp. salt-free garlic-pepper blend

4 low-sodium whole-wheat rolls

1. In a medium bowl, combine ground beef, onion, matzo meal, tomato sauce, and garlic-pepper blend. Mix well, and form into 4 (4-inch) patties.

2. Preheat a double-sided indoor grill. Cook burgers for 10 minutes or until the temperature on a food thermometer reads 160°F. Serve on whole-wheat rolls.

Salternative: If you prefer to prepare these burgers in the broiler, place patties on the rack of a broiler pan coated with nonstick cooking spray and broil on high 4 to 6 inches from the heat source for 6 to 8 minutes or until the temperature on a food thermometer reads 160°F, turning burgers halfway through cooking time.

PINCH OF SAGE

You can top your burger with your favorite additions—just be certain they aren't adding too much sodium. Use no-salt-added types of condiments, such as mustard and ketchup and any pickles or relish. If you make it a cheeseburger, choose a low-sodium slice.

Starters, Snacks, and Seasonings

In addition to eating three nutritious meals a day, you're going to want to nosh. Whether you're hosting a cocktail party, throwing a shower for a friend, or just lounging in front of the TV, you'll need some sodium-responsible options to enjoy. Hot hors d'oeuvres, satisfying snacks, favorite finger foods—they're delicious and refreshing when you need that between-meal pick-me-up.

Many of the foods we enjoy wouldn't be worth eating without the condiments, slathers, and seasonings that contribute their flavor. If you love fish dishes because of the great taste of tartar sauce or order a taco because you're in the mood for salsa, you'll appreciate the recipes in this part. You may be restricting sodium, but you certainly don't want to hold back flavor. All your sandwiches can be spread with zest, your main dishes can sing with the addition of a salsa or relish, and any savory recipe can be more appetizing when spiced up with an aromatic seasoning blend.

All-Occasion Appetizers

In This Chapter

- Lo-so light bites
- Keeping the serving size in mind
- Party perfect appetizers
- Sensational snack options

Most everyone loves nibbling on bite-size noshes, sampling a wide array of tasty tidbits. Appetizers whet your appetite for the coming meal, and because they're so small, they leave you hungry enough to eat it.

Of course, you may enjoy an entire meal made of an assortment of scrumptious little bites, Spanish *tapas* style. Keep in mind that all sodium and other nutritional tallies apply, even if you eat the food while you're standing.

Dainty delights also make great snacks. With their small size, appetizers naturally lend themselves to between-meal nibbling. And they're so versatile, you'll want to make them all the time!

Entertaining Ideas

Appetizers are such great all-around foods, what *can't* you do with them? From first-course offerings to cocktail party noshes, these little bites delight guests at every gathering.

If you'll be offering appetizers over a long period of time, keep safe food-handling in mind. Keep cold foods cold and hot foods hot. You can set cold dishes in bowls or trays filled with chipped ice to keep them at or below 40°F. Chafing dishes, warming trays, and slow cookers help keep cooked foods hot—at or above 140°F. Another option is to serve a small amount at a time. Exchange the plates instead of adding fresh morsels to those already sitting out. Discard any food left at room temperature for more than 2 hours. You want your guests to remember your fabulous party, not a resulting trip to the hospital.

> **PINCH OF SAGE**
>
> If you're hosting a hot, hot, hot party—and we mean *al fresco* in temperatures above 90°F—don't leave any foods out at room temperature more than 1 hour. Throw away any perishable foods you've held unrefrigerated for an hour or more.

Beware of Binging

Standing before a buffet spread with dozens of delectable tidbits may tempt you to pig out. So after you tuck your dangling tongue back in your mouth, survey the choices. Your stomach will be just as delighted with the noshes that are lower in sodium. Plus, you'll be proud of yourself for keeping your sodium level in check. Choosing hors d'oeuvres lower in sodium keeps you from feeling deprived.

If you just try each appetizer, you've probably reached the serving size. Eating more than one helping (and thereby more sodium) is too easy to do. Remember, a single helping of any appetizer is petite. They don't call them tidbits for nothing!

To Snack or Not to Snack?

Snacking is no longer a bad word. Eating a small serving between meals provides needed energy and keeps your blood sugar levels more consistent throughout the day. Also, you're less likely to grow hungry enough to binge when next you eat.

Appetizers are a convenient way to provide modest snacks. Choose wisely, and you can include a variety of foods for a well-balanced diet.

Cheddar Rice-Stuffed Mushrooms

A morsel of melted cheese with lightly seasoned rice is delivered in a tender mushroom cap.

Yield:	Prep time:	Cook time:	Serving size:
1 dozen mushroom caps	10 minutes	15 minutes	2 mushroom caps
Each serving has:			
88.1 calories	4.7 mg sodium		

1½ TB. unsalted butter

12 button mushrooms, stems removed and wiped with a damp paper towel

3 TB. sliced green onions

1 medium clove garlic, minced

½ cup cooked long-grain brown rice (about 3 TB. uncooked)

½ cup finely shredded low-sodium cheddar cheese

⅛ tsp. ground white pepper

1. Preheat the oven to 350°F.

2. In a small skillet over medium heat, melt ½ tablespoon butter. Add mushrooms, and cook, stirring, for 1 minute. Transfer mushrooms to a baking sheet, placing them gill side up.

3. In the same skillet over medium heat, melt remaining 1 tablespoon butter. Add green onions, and sauté for 1 minute. Add garlic, and sauté for 1 minute. Turn off heat, and stir in cooked brown rice. Place mixture into a small bowl, and let cool for a few minutes.

4. Stir cheddar cheese and white pepper into rice mixture, combining thoroughly. Spoon mixture into mushroom caps, mounding above hollows. Bake for 10 minutes or until cooked through and mushrooms start to exude liquid.

PINCH OF SAGE

If you have some extra stuffing mixture, you can spoon it into a few extra mushroom caps. Sautéing the mushroom caps helps them sit flat on the baking pan, but raw mushroom caps will cook during the baking time, too.

Icy Avocado Sorbet

This frozen treat is cool and creamy with a whisper of citrus.

Yield:	Prep time:	Freeze time:	Serving size:
6 servings	5 minutes	2 hours	3 small scoops
Each serving has:			
112 calories	6.9 mg sodium		

2 ripe avocados

Juice of 1 lemon

Juice of 1 lime

2 TB. water

1. Scoop avocado pulp into a food processor. Add lemon juice, lime juice, and water, and process for 20 seconds or until color is even and mixture is smooth.

2. Spoon mixture into a shallow dish. Cover with plastic wrap, and freeze for 30 minutes. Stir, cover, and freeze for 30 more minutes. Stir, cover, and freeze again until frozen.

3. Remove from the freezer at least 30 minutes before serving time. Use a small scoop or a melon baller to serve.

PINCH OF SAGE

Avocados discolor quickly, so don't cut into an avocado until you're ready to prepare it. The lemon and lime juices in this recipe help keep the avocado from browning.

Easy Cheddar Melt Potato Skins

Sink your teeth into these tasty baked potato skins filled with melty cheese and topped with mild green onions.

Yield:	Prep time:	Cook time:	Serving size:
8 potato halves	10 minutes	15 minutes	2 potato halves

Each serving has:	
214.9 calories	7.2 mg sodium

4 medium all-purpose potatoes	¼ cup chopped green onion tops
1 cup shredded *low-sodium* cheddar cheese	

1. Preheat the oven to 400°F. Spray a baking sheet with nonstick cooking spray.

2. Wash potatoes and prick all over with the tines of a fork. Arrange potatoes in a circle on a microwave-safe plate. Microwave on high for 10 to 12 minutes or until potatoes are tender. Remove potatoes from the microwave, cover with a paper towel, and let stand for 5 minutes.

3. Cut potatoes in half lengthwise. Using a spoon, scoop out pulp (reserve for making mashed potatoes or using as a thickening agent, as desired), leaving a thin ¼- to ½-inch shell.

4. Arrange potato skins on the prepared baking sheet. Sprinkle on cheddar cheese, and scatter green onions over top. Bake for 5 minutes or until cheese is melted and bubbly.

Salternative: You can serve these potato skins with your favorite tasty toppers, such as Fresh-Taste Tomato Salsa (recipe in Chapter 13), Great Guacamole (recipe in Chapter 10), and/or fat-free sour cream. Just remember to calculate in the additional sodium from the nutrition analysis or the nutrition facts label.

> **DEFINITION**
>
> **Low-sodium** denotes foods that contain 140 milligrams sodium or less per serving. Low-sodium cheddar cheese can actually be very low sodium with only 5 milligrams sodium per ounce. Because salt (sodium chloride) is integral in the production of cheese, low-sodium cheeses are made with the salt substitute potassium chloride instead, keeping the sodium content to a minimum.

Ricotta-Stuffed Cherry Tomatoes

Lightly seasoned smooth ricotta cheese adds a burst of flavor to these sweet tomato bites.

Yield:	Prep time:	Chill time:	Serving size:
18 tomatoes	15 minutes	30 minutes	2 tomatoes

Each serving has:	
30 calories	13.9 mg sodium

18 cherry tomatoes

$\frac{1}{2}$ cup *light-sodium* ricotta cheese

2 TB. chopped fresh basil

1 medium clove garlic, crushed

$\frac{1}{4}$ tsp. freshly ground black pepper

1. Slice off tops of cherry tomatoes, about $\frac{1}{4}$ the way down, with a sharp knife. Scoop out seeds using a small melon baller or a round $\frac{1}{4}$-teaspoon measuring spoon.

2. In a small bowl, combine ricotta cheese, basil, garlic, and pepper. Stir until evenly distributed.

3. Spoon into a snack-size sealable plastic bag, seal bag, and snip off a small piece of 1 corner. Pipe ricotta mixture into cherry tomatoes. Chill for 30 minutes before serving.

DEFINITION

Light sodium refers to a product that has less sodium than the regular version of that food—usually 50 percent less. Check the nutrition label for actual sodium amounts.

Thai Vegetable Stuffed Shells

A spicy sauced Asian vegetable medley with undertones of peanut butter is presented in a pasta shell.

Yield:	Prep time:	Cook time:	Serving size:
12 stuffed shells	5 minutes	15 minutes	2 stuffed shells
Each serving has:			
108.2 calories	15.1 mg sodium		

12 large pasta shells

1 cup thinly sliced carrots

1 cup small broccoli florets

1 cup coarsely chopped snow peas

2 TB. honey

1 TB. no-salt-added natural peanut butter

1 TB. Sodium-Wise Soy Sauce Stand-In (recipe in Chapter 12)

1 TB. chopped fresh cilantro

$\frac{1}{8}$ tsp. crushed red pepper flakes

1. Cook pasta shells according to the package directions. Drain and cool slightly.

2. Meanwhile, fill a steamer pot or a large saucepan with enough water to fall below the steamer basket when added, and bring to a boil over high heat. Add carrots, broccoli florets, and snow peas to a steamer basket, and place the basket in the pot or saucepan. Cover and steam vegetables over gently boiling water, reducing heat as necessary, for 5 to 7 minutes or until just tender.

3. In a medium bowl, whisk together honey, peanut butter, Sodium-Wise Soy Sauce Stand-In, cilantro, and crushed red pepper flakes until blended. Add vegetables to honey mixture, and stir until evenly coated.

4. To serve, spoon about 2 tablespoons vegetable mixture into each pasta shell. Serve warm or chilled as desired.

SALT PITFALL

Soy sauce is available in reduced-sodium versions, but even these options can add up to hundreds of milligrams sodium per small serving. If your diet allows for the extra sodium, you can substitute $\frac{1}{2}$ tablespoon reduced-sodium soy sauce in place of the 1 tablespoon Sodium-Wise Soy Sauce Stand-In called for in this recipe.

Creamy Mustard Deviled Eggs

Tangy yogurt mixes with homemade mustard to devil these hard-boiled eggs.

Yield:	Prep time:	Cook time:	Serving size:
1 dozen eggs	20 minutes	25 minutes	½ egg

Each serving has:			
52.1 calories	35.2 mg sodium		

6 large eggs

¼ cup fat-free plain yogurt

2 TB. Make-Your-Own Mustard
 (recipe in Chapter 12)

2 TB. white vinegar

Dash paprika

1. Place eggs in a medium saucepan, and cover with cold water. Cover the saucepan, and bring water to a boil over high heat. When water boils, remove the pan from heat. Let stand, covered, for 20 minutes. Immediately rinse eggs under cold water until cooled. Leave eggs immersed in cold water as you peel them.

2. Cut eggs in half lengthwise. Remove yolks to a small bowl, and mash with a fork until fine crumbs form. Add yogurt, Make-Your-Own Mustard, and white vinegar, and mix thoroughly.

3. Spoon yolk mixture into a snack-size sealable plastic bag, seal bag, and snip off a small piece of 1 corner. Pipe yolk mixture into egg whites, and lightly sprinkle paprika over tops for color. Chill before serving.

PINCH OF SAGE

Deviled eggs make great potluck dishes because you can prepare them the night before. For a pretty presentation, pipe the egg yolk mixture into the egg whites using a pastry bag with a fluted tip.

Flaming Pineapple Shrimp Skewers

Chili powder heats up these juicy pineapple and shrimp bites.

Yield:	Prep time:	Cook time:	Serving size:
10 skewers	10 minutes	2 minutes	1 skewer

Each serving has:			
81.4 calories	52.3 mg sodium		

½ lb. (about 20) medium tail-on
   shrimp, peeled and deveined,
   cooked or uncooked

1 (20-oz.) can pineapple chunks
   in their own juice, drained, and
   2 TB. juice reserved

1 tsp. Firehouse Chili Powder
   (recipe in Chapter 14) or other
   salt-free chili powder

2 TB. extra-virgin olive oil

2 medium cloves garlic, minced

1. In a medium bowl, place shrimp and pineapple chunks. Drizzle reserved pineapple juice over top, and toss to coat. Sprinkle on Firehouse Chili Powder, and toss again to coat.

2. In a large skillet over medium-high heat, heat extra-virgin olive oil and garlic. Add shrimp mixture, and sauté for 1 minute. Turn shrimp, and sauté for 1 more minute. Return to the bowl.

3. When cool enough to handle, thread pineapple and shrimp onto small wooden skewers, alternating pineapple and shrimp.

PINCH OF SAGE

To skewer shrimp, push the point of the skewer through the shrimp just above the tail and again near the head.

Italian-Style Stuffed New Potatoes

Waxy new potatoes are roasted with a pop of spinach and sun-dried tomatoes.

Yield:	Prep time:	Cook time:	Serving size:
1 dozen potatoes	20 minutes	30 minutes	2 potatoes
Each serving has:			
116.8 calories	59.9 mg sodium		

12 small new red potatoes (about 2-in. each)

4 dry-packed sun-dried tomatoes

¼ cup boiling water

1 cup packed baby spinach leaves

1 medium clove garlic, minced

1 medium green onion, finely chopped

1 TB. chopped fresh basil

¼ tsp. Salt-Shaker Substitute (recipe in Chapter 14) or other salt-free salt substitute seasoning blend

⅛ tsp. freshly ground black pepper

1 TB. chopped fresh Italian parsley

1. Fill a large saucepan with water, add potatoes, cover, and bring to a boil over high heat. Reduce heat to medium-low, and gently boil for 15 minutes or until just fork tender. Remove potatoes from the saucepan, and cool for 10 minutes or until cool enough to handle.

2. Preheat oven to 400°F. Spray a small baking sheet with nonstick cooking spray.

3. Meanwhile, place sun-dried tomatoes in a small bowl and pour boiling water over top. Soak for 5 minutes or until softened. Drain, reserving liquid. Chop sun-dried tomatoes, and set aside.

4. Heat a small nonstick skillet over medium heat. When hot, add reserved soaking liquid. Add spinach, and cook, stirring frequently, for 3 to 5 minutes or until wilted and much of liquid has evaporated.

5. Stir in garlic and green onion, and cook for 1 minute. Remove from heat and stir in sun-dried tomatoes, basil, Salt-Shaker Substitute, and pepper.

6. Using a melon baller or a small spoon, scoop out a small depression in each potato. Stir removed potato flesh with skin into spinach mixture until blended.

7. Spoon spinach mixture into depressions in potatoes, heaping up as needed to distribute evenly. Using a pastry brush, coat exposed areas of potatoes and stuffing with olive oil. Arrange on the prepared baking sheet, and bake for 10 minutes or until roasted.

8. To serve, place 2 stuffed potatoes on each serving plate. Sprinkle Italian parsley over tops. Serve with a dollop of sour cream, if desired.

> **PINCH OF SAGE**
>
> This recipe calls for red-skinned new potatoes because these less-mature potatoes are considered waxy and hold their shape when cooked. The skins are also thin. You could use any very small, thin-skinned new potatoes such as fingerlings instead.

Grilled Pizza-Parlor Quesadillas

Gooey mozzarella, lightly seasoned tomato sauce, and tasty toppings are all wrapped up in a toasted tortilla.

Yield:	Prep time:	Cook time:	Serving size:
2 (10-inch) quesadillas	10 minutes	16 minutes	2 wedges with 4 teaspoons sauce

Each serving has:		
262.6 calories	122.2 mg sodium	

1 (8-oz.) can no-salt-added tomato sauce

$\frac{1}{4}$ tsp. dried basil

$\frac{1}{8}$ tsp. dried oregano

$\frac{1}{8}$ tsp. garlic powder

$\frac{1}{8}$ tsp. onion powder

$\frac{1}{8}$ tsp. freshly ground black pepper

$\frac{1}{3}$ cup halved and sliced yellow onions

$\frac{1}{4}$ cup diced green bell peppers

4 medium button mushrooms, wiped with a damp paper towel, and trimmed and sliced

4 Fresh Tortillas (recipe in Chapter 19) or other low-sodium tortillas

$1\frac{1}{3}$ cups shredded fresh mozzarella cheese

1. In a small bowl, combine tomato sauce, basil, oregano, garlic powder, onion powder, and pepper. Stir to blend.

2. Spray a large, nonstick skillet with nonstick cooking spray. Add onions, green bell peppers, and mushrooms, and cook over medium heat for 3 or 4 minutes or until softened. Remove vegetables from the skillet, and set aside.

3. Spray the skillet with nonstick cooking spray again.

4. Spoon 2 tablespoons sauce over $\frac{1}{2}$ of each Fresh Tortilla. Sprinkle $\frac{1}{3}$ cup mozzarella cheese over sauce on each tortilla, and evenly distribute onion mixture over top. Fold over tortillas, and add to the skillet. Cook, 1 at a time, over medium heat for 2 minutes on each side or until toasted and cheese is melted. Let each quesadilla stand briefly before cutting into 3 wedges to serve.

5. Heat remaining sauce to serve as a dip for quesadillas.

 PINCH OF SAGE

Use a pizza cutter to make quick work of slicing the quesadillas.

Delicious Dips and Scoops

In This Chapter

- Super low-sodium dips
- Serving party-friendly dips
- Responsible snacking suggestions
- Tips for watching the serving size

One sure way to draw a crowd is to bring out a dip. Everyone gathers 'round, and conversation and laughter are sure to follow.

Dips may also be a snacking solution. You know you should eat more fruits and vegetables, but plain-Jane slices don't do it for you. A dip can get you munching and crunching your fruits and veggies with delight. With the dips and scoops recipes in this chapter, you can get a great fresh taste without excessive sodium. Let the dipping begin!

Throwing a "Scooper" Party

What's a party without a dip or two—or three? To throw a "scooper" party, you just need to eye the dip from a guest's perspective.

Make the dip easily accessible in bowls close to where the action is—your guests won't have to stretch to reach the dip, and you'll have less mess to clean up after the party. Refill the dip, as well as the dippers, for happy guests and safety purposes. Foods shouldn't sit out for more than 2 hours; putting out smaller portions more frequently is a good idea. And if your dippers require toothpicks, provide a place for your revelers to dispose of them. You don't even want to think of what they may do with them otherwise.

Smart Dipping

When you're browsing the dip buffet or making yourself a snack, remember, dips are intended to complement the dippers, not overpower them. Be aware of serving size, and don't use a full serving on a single apple slice! If you decide to eat more, remember to count the additional sodium, calories, fat, and so on.

Dips do make good snacks and many times enable you to eat more good-for-you fruits and vegetables. But you don't want to munch thoughtlessly in front of the TV. Hitting the bottom of the bowl is not a good indicator of when to stop eating. If you're apt to eat your way through a whole bowl of dip, place just one portion on a plate.

SALT PITFALL

Many great dips are traditionally served with high-sodium dippers such as salted chips, pretzels, crackers, and breads. Be sure your dippers don't spoil the reduced sodium of the dip. Fresh fruits and veggies make great dipping vehicles. Otherwise, try unsalted chips, pretzels, crackers, and low-sodium breads.

The High Price of Convenience

Picking up a carton of chip dip at the supermarket seems so easy. Now that you know the importance of reading nutrition labels, though, you'll notice the high sodium content of most commercially prepared dips and envelopes of dip mixes. But that doesn't mean you have to throw down your carrot stick or resign yourself to eating everything plain and dry from now on.

If you crave the convenience of a commercial dip mix, you can buy a small selection of low-sodium packets. But making homemade dips and scoops that are lower in sodium is so easy. You can readily purchase ingredients at most supermarkets, and preparation is, many times, quick and simple. Plus, the taste is fresher. Easy, better-tasting, and good-for-you: get ready to plunge that carrot stick into a concoction of luscious proportion!

Zippy Jalapeño Hummus

Traditional hummus seasonings of garlic and cumin are enhanced by the mild spiciness of jalapeños.

Yield:	Prep time:	Serving size:
1 cup	5 minutes	2 tablespoons

Each serving has:		
53.8 calories	0.5 mg sodium	

1 (15-oz.) can no-salt-added chickpeas, drained (2 TB. liquid reserved)

3 medium fresh jalapeño peppers, ribs and seeds removed, and chopped

3 medium cloves garlic, minced

$\frac{1}{2}$ tsp. ground cumin

2 TB. fresh lemon juice

1. In a blender or food processor, combine chickpeas, jalapeño peppers, garlic, cumin, lemon juice, and reserved chickpea liquid.

2. Blend on high speed for 1 minute or until smooth, stopping to scrape down the sides as necessary. Serve with low-sodium pita bread, crackers, or your favorite veggies.

SALT PITFALL

After seeding and chopping the jalapeño peppers, be sure to wash your hands. If you forget and then touch your eyes or lips, you'll find out the hard way that the essence carries the heat of the peppers.

Lemon-Fresh Mediterranean White Bean Dip

Brightened by the citrus burst of lemon, smooth white beans are seasoned with garlic and *Italian parsley*.

Yield:	Prep time:	Serving size:
1¾ cups	10 minutes	2 tablespoons
Each serving has:		
58.2 calories	1.1 mg sodium	

3 TB. extra-virgin olive oil

2 medium cloves garlic, sliced

¼ cup packed Italian parsley leaves

2 cups cooked Great Northern or other white beans, drained

2 TB. fresh lemon juice

1 tsp. Salt-Shaker Substitute (recipe in Chapter 14) or other salt-free salt substitute seasoning blend or more to taste

¼ tsp. freshly ground black pepper

1. Heat a small skillet over medium-low heat. When hot, add extra-virgin olive oil, and heat for 1 minute. Add garlic, and cook for 1 minute or until fragrant.

2. Add Italian parsley and Great Northern beans, and cook, stirring, for 1 minute. Remove from heat.

3. In a food processor, combine bean mixture, lemon juice, Salt-Shaker Substitute, and pepper. Cover and process for 90 seconds, stopping to scrape down the sides as needed. Serve at room temperature, or heat to serve warm, as desired.

DEFINITION

Italian parsley is also known as flat-leaf parsley and tends to be more flavorful than curly leaf parsley.

Great Guacamole

The richness of avocado carries tangy tomatoes and spicy jalapeños.

Yield:	Prep time:	Serving size:
1⅓ cups	10 minutes	2 tablespoons

Each serving has:		
33.6 calories	2.7 mg sodium	

1 medium ripe avocado, halved and pitted

1 TB. fresh lemon juice

1 TB. fresh lime juice

1 medium clove garlic, minced

1 small tomato, finely diced

1 medium fresh jalapeño pepper, ribs and seeds removed, and minced

1. Using a metal spoon, scoop avocado pulp out of peel and place in a medium glass bowl. Add lemon juice and lime juice, and stir and chop avocado to blend.

2. Add garlic, tomato, and jalapeño pepper, and stir until blended and desired consistency is reached. Serve immediately or chill briefly.

PINCH OF SAGE

To remove the pit from an avocado, cut the avocado in half. Embed the middle of the knife blade into the pit, and slowly turn the knife to release the pit.

Mediterranean Roasted Eggplant Dip

The deep flavor of roasted eggplants is brightened by mint and toasted almonds.

Yield:	Prep time:	Cook time:	Serving size:
3½ cups	10 minutes plus 40 minutes rest time	1 hour	2 tablespoons

Each serving has:	
22.2 calories	4.7 mg sodium

2 medium eggplants	1½ TB. fresh lemon juice
⅔ cup fat-free plain yogurt	⅛ tsp. freshly ground black pepper
4 medium cloves garlic, minced	4 tsp. dried mint
½ medium fresh jalapeño pepper, minced	½ cup chopped unsalted almonds, toasted
1 tsp. ground cumin	

1. Preheat the oven to 400°F.

2. Place eggplants on a baking sheet, and prick all over with the tines of a fork. Bake for 1 hour or until tender, turning occasionally. Let cool.

3. Peel eggplants, and place pulp in a colander over the sink to drain for 30 minutes.

4. Transfer eggplants to a food processor, and pulse for 10 seconds or until puréed. Add yogurt, garlic, jalapeño pepper, cumin, lemon juice, pepper, and mint, and pulse for 15 to 20 seconds or until thoroughly blended.

5. Cover and chill eggplant mixture for up to 8 hours, if needed. Just before serving, fold in almonds. Serve with low-sodium pita chips, your favorite veggies, or unsalted crackers.

PINCH OF SAGE

To toast almonds, place them in a dry skillet over medium heat for 2 to 5 minutes, watching them carefully and shaking occasionally to avoid burning.

Creamy Strawberry Fruit Dip

Smooth and dreamy, this dip softens the tang of yogurt with sweet whipped topping.

Yield:	Prep time:	Serving size:
3½ cups	5 minutes	2 tablespoons

Each serving has:		
32 calories	5.5 mg sodium	

1 (8-oz.) container frozen whipped topping, thawed

1 (6-oz.) container low-fat strawberry yogurt or your favorite flavor

1. In a medium bowl, stir together whipped topping and yogurt until thoroughly combined.

2. Serve with your favorite fresh fruits.

SALT PITFALL

You may substitute low-fat or fat-free whipped topping in this recipe. It will add a small amount of sodium to each serving, though. Check the nutrition labels for specific information.

Crisp and Creamy Waldorf Dip

Offer this fruity and chunky dip to your guests who love the classic Waldorf medley of apples, grapes, and walnuts.

Yield:	Prep time:	Serving size:
3 cups	15 minutes	¼ cup

Each serving has:		
70.7 calories	11.7 mg sodium	

1 cup fat-free plain yogurt

2 TB. honey

1 TB. fresh lemon juice

1½ cups finely diced McIntosh apples (about 1 very large apple)

1 cup sliced seedless red grapes

½ cup chopped unsalted walnuts

1. In a medium bowl, combine yogurt, honey, and lemon juice. Stir until blended.

2. Add apples into yogurt mixture, and stir to coat. Add grapes and walnuts, and stir to distribute evenly. Serve immediately, or chill for up to 4 hours. Serve with celery sticks, apple slices, or low-sodium crackers or pita chips, as desired.

Lemon Lover's Poppy Seed Dip

Honey-sweetened sour cream packs the tart punch of lemon.

Yield:	Prep time:	Chill time:	Serving size:
14 tablespoons	5 minutes	30 minutes	2 tablespoons

Each serving has:			
41 calories	18 mg sodium		

⅔ cup fat-free sour cream

4 tsp. honey

1 tsp. finely grated lemon zest

1 TB. fresh lemon juice

1 TB. poppy seeds

1. In a small bowl, stir together sour cream and honey. Stir in lemon zest and lemon juice, followed by poppy seeds, until evenly distributed.

2. Cover and chill for at least 30 minutes before serving. Serve with apple slices, seedless green grapes, or your other favorite fruits.

PINCH OF SAGE

To keep honey from clinging to your measuring spoon, first spray the measuring spoon with a little nonstick cooking spray. The honey will slide right out, especially if your measuring spoon is metal.

Green Herbed Veggie Dip

This yogurt-based dip is seasoned with sweet marjoram and parsley with minced fresh garlic.

Yield:	Prep time:	Serving size:
½ cup	5 minutes	2 tablespoons
Each serving has:		
16.6 calories	18.7 mg sodium	

½ cup fat-free plain yogurt

2 cloves garlic, minced

4 tsp. dried parsley flakes

¼ tsp. dried marjoram

¼ tsp. freshly ground black pepper

¼ tsp. onion powder

1. In a small bowl, combine yogurt, garlic, parsley flakes, marjoram, pepper, and onion powder. Stir until blended.

2. Serve with your favorite veggie dippers.

Fiesta Black Bean Dip

Keep this dip on hand to satisfy your craving for a mingling of favorite Mexican flavors—beans and tomatoes splashed with lime.

Yield:	Prep time:	Chill time:	Serving size:
3 cups	10 minutes	1 hour	2 tablespoons
Each serving has:			
13.7 calories	39.7 mg sodium		

1 (15-oz.) can *no-salt-added* black
   beans, rinsed and drained

2 TB. fresh lime juice

1 medium clove garlic, crushed

½ cup diced tomatoes, seeded as
   desired

¼ cup sliced green onions

½ cup fat-free plain yogurt

¼ tsp. ground cayenne

1. In a medium bowl, and using a fork, mash black beans with lime juice and garlic.

2. Add tomatoes, green onions, yogurt, and cayenne, and stir until blended.

3. Cover and chill for at least 1 hour before serving. Serve with carrot sticks, bell pepper strips, or unsalted baked tortilla chips.

DEFINITION

Foods with **no-salt-added** labels have been processed without introduced salt where they typically would be prepared with salt. Nutrition labels will list sodium amounts for individual servings.

Snack-Time Finger Foods

In This Chapter

- Sin-free low-sodium snacks
- Snacking without feeling deprived
- In-between meal munchies
- Fitting snacks into your daily eating plan

Now that you're all grown up and following a low-sodium diet, you have to behave appropriately—eat bland foods, shun anything that tastes good, always use utensils, right? Not so! If you make good snack choices—and plenty of delicious options are awaiting you—food can still be fun.

Getting the munchies is inevitable, so plan accordingly. Have your favorite snacks on hand, and toss that silverware! These hunger-busters are for fingers only.

Snack Attack Flak

Once upon a time, snackers were thought to be weak creatures who lacked the willpower of prudent eaters who held fast to the institution of three meals a day. Fortunately, now snacking is not only an accepted but also an encouraged affair.

Naturally, you can't run rampant with this newfound notion. Portion control is essential, and sodium control is especially crucial. If you're a bottom-of-the-bag muncher, take out only a single serving. Dividing recipe yields into single portions helps you keep a snack attack from overpowering your low-sodium efforts.

If you're apt to hit the vending machine, plan out your snacks. A little preparation keeps you in control of your sodium consumption.

Sensible snacks can add essential variety to your diet. Look at your snack as a little pick-me-up that offers nutrition and fuel to push you on to your next full meal.

Of course, if you don't have time to whip up any of these snacks, fresh fruits and veggies always make a smart snack choice. You can't go wrong with a banana or carrot sticks.

> **PINCH OF SAGE**
>
> Just a glance at the nutrition label on many bagged snacks tells you they're swimming in sodium. Potato chips, corn chips, pretzels, popcorn, crackers, and the rest aren't intended for the lo-so crowd. Rather than totally cut out snacking, however, buy reduced-sodium alternatives. Be sure to check the labels for sodium amounts. Or prepare your own alternatives with the recipes in this chapter!

Peanut Butter–Banana Swirls

Creamy peanut butter and sweet banana are wrapped up in a tender tortilla.

Yield:	Prep time:	Serving size:
16 swirls	5 minutes	4 swirls
Each serving has:		
65.2 calories	0 mg sodium	

¼ cup no-salt-added natural peanut butter

2 Fresh Tortillas (recipe in Chapter 19) or other low-sodium tortillas

1 medium ripe banana, peeled

1. Spread peanut butter over Fresh Tortillas.

2. Mash banana with a fork, and spread over peanut butter.

3. Roll up tortillas tightly. Cut 1-inch slices on the diagonal.

> **PINCH OF SAGE**
>
> Keep the tortilla whole, and this recipe also makes a delicious lunchtime sandwich.

Italian-Seasoned Popcorn

Basil and oregano season this light popped corn snack.

Yield:	Prep time:	Cook time:	Serving size:
8 cups	5 minutes	5 minutes	2 cups
Each serving has:			
123.4 calories	1.4 mg sodium		

¼ cup popcorn kernels	½ tsp. dried oregano
3 TB. unsalted butter, melted	¼ tsp. garlic powder
½ tsp. dried basil	¼ tsp. onion powder

1. In a hot-air popcorn machine, pop popcorn kernels.

2. In a small bowl, stir together melted butter, basil, oregano, garlic powder, and onion powder. Drizzle over popcorn, and toss to coat.

PINCH OF SAGE

If you don't have a hot-air popcorn machine, prepare the popcorn as you usually do. If you add oil, remember to add that information to the nutritional analysis. And if you're watching your fat or caloric intake, you can spray the popcorn with a sodium-free buttery spray and then toss with the seasonings.

Baked Garlic Pita Chips

These substantial chips provide a wheaty crunch with a hint of garlic.

Yield:	Prep time:	Cook time:	Serving size:
2 dozen chips	10 minutes	8 minutes	6 chips
Each serving has:			
153.3 calories	2 mg sodium		

4 Mini Wheat Pita Pockets (recipe in Chapter 19)	1 TB. extra-virgin olive oil
	¼ tsp. garlic powder

1. Preheat the oven to 375°F.

2. Cut each Mini Wheat Pita Pocket into 6 wedges, and arrange in a single layer on a large baking sheet.

3. In a small bowl, whisk together extra-virgin olive oil and garlic powder. Using a pastry brush, lightly coat both sides of each wedge with olive oil mixture completely.

4. Bake for 8 minutes or until golden-brown, turning over each wedge halfway through baking time. Cool on the baking sheet on a wire rack before serving.

Salternative: If your pita pockets are well puffed, you can prepare thinner chips by cutting each half into wedges. Bake just until crisp.

PINCH OF SAGE

Remember that recipes are really guidelines and seasonings can—and should—be adjusted to suit your tastes and needs. Personalize your baked pita chips by adding your favorite dried herbs and spices to the olive oil.

¡Olé! Taco Popcorn

Coat your next bowl of popcorn with the spicy kick of hot peppers and cumin.

Yield:	Prep time:	Cook time:	Serving size:
8 cups	5 minutes	5 minutes	2 cups
Each serving has:			
148.2 calories	2 mg sodium		

¼ cup popcorn kernels
¼ cup unsalted butter, melted

¾ tsp. Taco Seasoning Mix (recipe in Chapter 14)

1. Pour popcorn kernels into a hot-air popcorn machine and pop.

2. In a small bowl, stir together melted butter and Taco Seasoning Mix. Drizzle over popcorn, and toss to coat.

PINCH OF SAGE

The recipe for Taco Seasoning Mix has a bit of a kick to it. If you prefer the milder taste of another salt-free taco seasoning mix, you may substitute it in this recipe. The same goes for a more fiery blend. Read the ingredients list carefully, though; most commercial blends contain sodium.

Sugar-and-Spice Pecans

Toasted mild pecans are sweetened and coated with rich fall baking spices.

Yield:	Prep time:	Cook time:	Serving size:
3 cups	10 minutes	20 minutes	¼ cup
Each serving has:			
328 calories	2.5 mg sodium		

6 TB. unsalted butter	1 TB. ground cinnamon
3 cups unsalted pecan halves	1 TB. ground cloves
1½ cups confectioners' sugar	1 TB. ground nutmeg

1. In a large, heavy skillet over low to medium-low heat, melt butter. Add pecans, and stir to coat. Cook, stirring occasionally, for 20 minutes or until heated through and lightly toasted. Using a slotted spoon, remove pecans to a paper towel–lined plate.

2. Meanwhile, place confectioners' sugar, cinnamon, cloves, and nutmeg in a large zipper-lock bag. Seal the bag, and shake until blended.

3. Add pecans to the bag, and shake until evenly coated. Pour pecans into a colander over the sink, and shake to remove excess confectioners' sugar mixture. Spread pecans in a single layer on a sheet of waxed paper, and allow to cool completely before storing in an airtight container.

PINCH OF SAGE

If you don't have a colander, you can remove the coated pecans from the bag with a slotted spoon, shaking off the excess confectioners' sugar mixture.

Vinegared Cucumbers

Crisp cucumbers are infused with the tart taste of vinegar.

Yield:	Prep time:	Chill time:	Serving size:
2 cups	5 minutes	30 minutes	½ cup

Each serving has:		
14 calories	2.6 mg sodium	

1 large cucumber, peeled and sliced	1⅓ cups water
	⅔ cup white vinegar

1. Place cucumber in a medium bowl. Pour water and white vinegar over top.

2. Cover and chill for at least 30 minutes.

Salternative: You may add onion slices to the mixture, if you like.

Sweet and Crunchy Trail Mix

This trail mix is a sweet jumble of nuts, seeds, dried berries, and chocolate.

Yield:	Prep time:	Serving size:
2 cups	5 minutes	½ cup

Each serving has:	
364 calories	5 mg sodium

¼ cup unsalted dry-roasted peanuts	¼ cup raisins
¼ cup unsalted whole almonds	¼ cup dried cranberries
¼ cup unsalted cashew pieces	¼ cup dried cherries
¼ cup unsalted sunflower seeds	¼ cup semisweet chocolate chips

1. In a large bowl, combine peanuts, almonds, cashew pieces, sunflower seeds, raisins, cranberries, cherries, and chocolate chips.

2. Divide into individual portions, place in zipper-lock bags, and grab whenever a snack craving hits.

PINCH OF SAGE

You can substitute any of your favorite unsalted nuts, seeds, or dried fruits in this easily adaptable recipe. Try walnuts, pecans, macadamia nuts, soy nuts, pumpkin seeds, dried pineapple, dried papaya, dates, banana chips, and more. Stored tightly sealed in a cool, dry place, your mix will keep until the earliest "best by" date stamped on your individual ingredients.

Pan-Fried Zucchini Rounds

Tender zucchini get a crisp breading flavored with a sprinkle of garlic powder.

Yield:	Prep time:	Cook time:	Serving size:
1 cup	10 minutes	20 minutes	¼ cup
Each serving has:			
145.9 calories	17.3 mg sodium		

1 large egg

¼ cup whole-wheat flour

¼ tsp. freshly ground black pepper

3 TB. extra-virgin olive oil

1 medium zucchini, sliced

¼ tsp. garlic powder or to taste

1. In a small bowl, beat egg.

2. In another small, shallow bowl, stir together whole-wheat flour and pepper.

3. In a nonstick skillet over medium to medium-low heat, heat 1 tablespoon extra-virgin olive oil.

4. Dip zucchini slices into egg and then dredge in seasoned flour to coat, shaking off excess. Add to the skillet, and fry for 3 minutes or until browned. Turn and fry for 3 more minutes or until underside is browned. (You may have to cook zucchini in batches. Add more extra-virgin olive oil to the skillet as necessary.) Using a slotted spoon, remove zucchini to a paper towel–lined plate.

5. Sprinkle on garlic powder.

Salternative: If you think these zucchini slices need a bit more seasoning, sprinkle on your favorite salt-free salt substitute seasoning blend.

PINCH OF SAGE

If you have leftover tomato sauce from the Individual Lasagna Casseroles recipe in Chapter 18, use it as a dipping sauce for these Pan-Fried Zucchini Rounds.

Cheddar and Jalapeño Nachos

Crisp and crunchy tortilla chips are drenched in smooth cheese sauce and hot jalapeño slices.

Yield:	Prep time:	Cook time:	Serving size:
2 servings	5 minutes	3 minutes	18 tortilla chips with 3 tablespoons cheese sauce and $\frac{1}{2}$ jalapeño pepper

Each serving has:	
224.5 calories	19.1 mg sodium

1 tsp. cornstarch

$\frac{1}{4}$ cup fat-free milk

$\frac{1}{4}$ cup finely shredded low-sodium cheddar cheese

3 doz. small *unsalted* baked tortilla chips (2 servings)

1 medium fresh jalapeño pepper, ribs and seeds removed, and thinly sliced

1. In a small saucepan, whisk cornstarch into milk until blended. Heat over medium heat just until bubbles form around edge of the pan, and reduce heat to low. Slowly whisk in cheddar cheese until melted and smooth. Remove from heat.

2. Arrange tortilla chips on 2 plates, and pour cheese sauce over chips. Scatter jalapeño pepper slices over each portion, and serve.

DEFINITION

When a food's labeled **unsalted,** it means no salt was added during processing, where it typically would have been. As with the term *no-salt-added,* foods labeled *unsalted* may contain sodium. Read the nutrition label to find out how much.

Ants on a Log

Sweet raisins and creamy peanut butter are delivered in crunchy celery sticks kids of all ages will love.

Yield:	Prep time:	Serving size:
1 serving	5 minutes	4 logs

Each serving has:		
262 calories	63.6 mg sodium	

2 TB. no-salt-added natural peanut butter	4 (3-in.) celery sticks
	2 TB. raisins

1. Spread peanut butter on celery sticks.

2. Push raisins into top of peanut butter.

SALT PITFALL

Celery is one vegetable that is comparatively high in sodium. Try to limit it in your diet.

Classic Condiments

In This Chapter

- Enjoying your favorite condiments without excessive sodium
- Preparing your own low-sodium spreads and sauces
- Adding flavor without adding sodium
- Enhancing foods, not overpowering them

Do you find yourself craving fish because you fancy tartar sauce? Do people question if you'd like a little burger with your mustard? If so, you know how powerful a condiment can be in imparting delectable flavor to your favorite foods.

Many of the classic condiments are high in sodium. Maybe you've found suitable alternatives available at your local supermarket, or perhaps you've discovered a mail-order supplier that keeps you stocked up on your favorites. If not, you do have options.

You can easily prepare many spreads and sauces at home. If you've been dying for a bowl of navy beans seasoned with a heaping teaspoon of horseradish or a finger-licking barbecue chicken leg, you've come to the right place. Fresh condiments you prepare yourself can satisfy your taste buds and let you enjoy your favorite foods again—without ruining your low-sodium resolve.

Homespun Yum

Many of your favorite condiments are now available commercially in no-salt-added and low-sodium versions, but you still may find it difficult to come by some of them. If you don't have access to sodium-responsible spreads and sauces, you don't have to do without.

Making condiments at home can be convenient. You can always have freshly prepared, great-tasting accompaniments when you need them. If you make fresh tartar sauce, you certainly won't be disappointed to find that the bottle of tartar sauce in the refrigerator expired 3 months ago. You can mix up what you'll use the very night you're cooking seafood.

> **PINCH OF SAGE**
>
> If you can't convince your local supermarket to stock your favorite condiment in a no-salt-added, sodium-free, or low-sodium version, and you prefer not to make your own (but these recipes are easy, really!), check out the additional resources we've provided at idiotsguides.com/lowsodiumcooking for more information on mail-order sources.

Another benefit of homemade condiments is the savings. The ingredients are inexpensive. You'll be liberated from purchasing large quantities of a condiment to use only a quarter of it before it goes bad.

The top advantage, of course, is that you control the sodium. Homemade condiments allow you to enjoy the good taste without giving in to the temptation to eat too much sodium in favor of flavor.

Using a Light Hand

Spreads or sauces added to your sandwiches, meats, soups, salads, eggs, vegetables, and more should add flavor, and that's all. Even if the condiments are low in sodium, you don't want to use a heavy hand, piling on additional calories and fat.

Be sure to note the serving sizes. A single serving of a condiment is intended to enhance your food, not overpower it. You *can* have too much of a good thing!

Homemade Horseradish

With just two ingredients, the piquant taste of fresh horseradish root powers through.

Yield:	Prep time:	Serving size:
1 cup	10 minutes	1 teaspoon
Each serving has:		
3 calories	0.5 mg sodium	

1 cup pared, coarsely chopped horseradish root   ½ cup white vinegar

1. In a well-ventilated area (gas mask optional), place horseradish root in a blender. Chop on high speed for a few seconds. Carefully tip up the lid's cap to pour in white vinegar a little at a time while blending. Chop for 2 minutes or until mixture is creamy, stopping to scrape down the sides as necessary.

2. Pack into small glass jars with tight-fitting lids, and refrigerate for up to 3 or 4 months.

PINCH OF SAGE

This is a quick, easy way to save on the salt and other added ingredients in many commercially prepared horseradish sauces. Use the amount of vinegar necessary to make the horseradish mixture creamy.

Make-Your-Own Mustard

With its super-low-sodium content, you can enjoy this smooth sauce with a bit of a bite.

Yield:	Prep time:	Cook time:	Serving size:
½ cup	5 minutes	10 minutes	1 teaspoon
Each serving has:			
22.5 calories	2.8 mg sodium		

¼ cup dry mustard   ⅓ cup cider vinegar

⅓ cup granulated sugar   1 large egg

1. In the top of a double boiler, combine dry mustard, sugar, cider vinegar, and egg. Whisk together until very smooth.

2. Cook, stirring constantly, over simmering water for 10 minutes or until well thickened.

3. Pour into a clean jar, and let cool completely. Cover with a tight-fitting lid, and store in the refrigerator for 3 to 5 days.

PINCH OF SAGE

If you don't have a double boiler, you can use two heavy pans if one sits nicely in the top of the other. Combine the mixture in the top pan off the heat while you bring the water in the bottom pan to a simmer on the burner. Keep the water in the bottom pan just at a simmer while cooking the mustard.

Easy BBQ Sauce

This tomato-based sauce is sweet and savory.

Yield:	Prep time:	Serving size:
2¼ cups	15 minutes	2 tablespoons
Each serving has:		
34.2 calories	3.7 mg sodium	

1 cup no-salt-added ketchup	1 TB. minced green bell pepper
1 cup water	2 tsp. dry mustard
2 TB. firmly packed light brown sugar	1 tsp. Salt-Shaker Substitute (recipe in Chapter 14) or other salt-free salt-substitute seasoning blend
2 tsp. fresh lemon juice	
2 TB. unsalted butter, melted	1 tsp. celery seeds
2 TB. minced yellow onions	

1. In a medium stainless-steel or glass bowl, combine ketchup, water, light brown sugar, lemon juice, butter, onions, green bell pepper, dry mustard, Salt-Shaker Substitute, and celery seeds.

2. Whisk until well blended. If not using immediately, refrigerate tightly covered for up to 4 days.

Salternative: You can reduce or increase this barbecue sauce as needed for your favorite recipes.

PINCH OF SAGE

The dried seed of the celery plant may be tiny, but it packs a powerful punch of flavor. Use a light hand whenever adding celery seeds to your cooking.

Like-So for Mayo

This spread is tangier than mayonnaise, but it adds a nice zing to your favorite sandwiches.

Yield:	Prep time:	Serving size:
2 teaspoons	1 minute	2 teaspoons
Each serving has:		
12.1 calories	5.3 mg sodium	

1 tsp. fat-free plain yogurt	1 tsp. fat-free sour cream

1. In a small bowl, stir together yogurt and sour cream until blended.

2. Spread onto a sandwich as desired.

 PINCH OF SAGE

Check the sell-by date on both yogurt and sour cream to ensure freshness. After opening, store tightly covered for up to 1 week. To prolong freshness after opening, store the tightly covered container upside down to minimize air exposure. You may double the shelf life for use, but always check for spoilage before using.

Home-Style Mustard

This mildly tangy, lightly sweetened mustard pairs well with herbal additions.

Yield:	Prep time:	Cook time:	Serving size:
½ cup	5 minutes	15 minutes	2 teaspoons
Each serving has:			
44.3 calories	8.1 mg sodium		

¼ cup white vinegar	6 TB. firmly packed light brown sugar
3 TB. dry mustard	1 large egg
2 TB. water	

1. In a small saucepan over high heat, whisk together white vinegar and dry mustard. Add water, light brown sugar, and egg, and whisk to combine. Cook, whisking constantly, for 5 minutes or until bubbles appear around edges.

2. When bubbles appear, reduce heat as needed to maintain a simmer. Gently simmer, whisking, for 10 minutes.

3. Pour into a clean jar, and let cool. Cover and refrigerate tightly covered for 3 to 5 days.

Salternative: If you want to gussy-up this mustard, add your choice of chopped fresh or dried herbs to taste. Try basil, dill, tarragon, cilantro, rosemary, for starters.

Kitchen Ketchup

Thick and rich, this sweet and spicy tomato ketchup fills the bill.

Yield:	Prep time:	Cook time:	Serving size:
3 cups	15 minutes	4 hours, 10 minutes	1 tablespoon
Each serving has:			
23.7 calories	10.9 mg sodium		

3 (6-oz.) cans no-salt-added tomato paste

4 cups water

$\frac{1}{2}$ cup chopped yellow onions

$\frac{1}{2}$ cup chopped celery

$\frac{1}{2}$ cup cider vinegar

$\frac{1}{2}$ cup granulated sugar

2 TB. unsalted butter

1 TB. firmly packed light brown sugar

1 tsp. molasses

$\frac{1}{8}$ tsp. freshly ground black pepper

$\frac{1}{8}$ tsp. garlic powder

$\frac{1}{8}$ tsp. onion powder

$\frac{1}{8}$ tsp. dried basil

$\frac{1}{8}$ tsp. dried tarragon

$\frac{1}{8}$ tsp. ground cinnamon

$\frac{1}{8}$ tsp. ground cloves

1. In a food processor, combine tomato paste, water, onions, celery, cider vinegar, and sugar. Process for 1 or 2 minutes or until smooth. (Process in batches if your food processor isn't large enough to hold all the ingredients.) Pour mixture into a large saucepan set over medium heat.

2. Add butter, light brown sugar, molasses, pepper, garlic powder, onion powder, basil, tarragon, cinnamon, and cloves to the saucepan. Bring to a simmer, reduce heat as needed to maintain a simmer, and gently simmer, uncovered and stirring occasionally, for 4 hours or until thickened, reduced, and deep red.

3. Pour ketchup into tightly covered containers, and refrigerate for up to 1 month.

PINCH OF SAGE

If you can't find no-salt-added tomato paste, you can use regular tomato paste. The difference in sodium content is negligible at about 15 milligrams of sodium per serving versus 20 milligrams in the regular stuff.

Dilly Tartar Sauce

After one taste of this fresh dill-infused sauce, you'll happily toss out the high-sodium bottled stuff.

Yield:	Prep time:	Serving size:
⁷⁄₈ cup	10 minutes	2 tablespoons
Each serving has:		
14.4 calories	11.7 mg sodium	

¼ cup fat-free plain yogurt

¼ cup fat-free sour cream

¼ cup minced yellow onions

3 TB. finely chopped fresh dill

¼ tsp. ground white pepper

1. In a small bowl, combine yogurt, sour cream, onions, dill, and white pepper. Stir until thoroughly blended.

2. Cover and refrigerate if not serving immediately, and use within 2 days.

Salternative: You may decrease or increase this recipe as needed.

Sodium-Wise Soy Sauce Stand-In

Rich-bodied with a depth of flavor from the molasses and sesame seed oil, this sauce makes a good mild soy sauce substitute.

Yield:	Prep time:	Cook time:	Serving size:
¾ cup	2 minutes	15 minutes	1 tablespoon
Each serving has:			
12 calories	24.1 mg sodium		

1½ cups unsalted beef stock	⅛ tsp. garlic powder
½ cup red wine vinegar	⅛ tsp. ground ginger
1 TB. molasses	⅛ tsp. freshly ground black pepper
1 tsp. sesame seed oil	

1. In a small saucepan over medium heat, stir together beef stock, red wine vinegar, molasses, sesame seed oil, garlic powder, ginger, and pepper. Bring to a simmer, and reduce heat as needed to maintain a simmer for 5 minutes, stirring occasionally. Let cool.

2. Pour into a clean jar, and let cool. Cover and refrigerate tightly covered for 1 or 2 months.

PINCH OF SAGE

Stocking a wide variety of flavorful vinegars is easy. Stored tightly covered in a cool, dark place, vinegars keep indefinitely.

Sun-Up Tomato Gravy

Lightly sweetened and slightly thickened, this sauce stars the juicy goodness of tomatoes.

Yield:	Prep time:	Cook time:	Serving size:
1¼ cups	5 minutes	20 minutes	¼ cup
Each serving has:			
45.2 calories	34.8 mg sodium		

1 (14.5-oz.) can no-salt-added diced tomatoes, with juice	1½ TB. water
1½ TB. all-purpose flour	2 TB. firmly packed light brown sugar

1. In a medium saucepan over medium heat, bring tomatoes and juice to a boil, stirring occasionally. Reduce heat to medium-low, and stir. Return tomatoes to a boil.

2. Meanwhile, in a small bowl, whisk together flour and water.

3. When tomatoes are boiling, stir in flour mixture and light brown sugar. Cook, stirring, for 10 to 15 minutes or until smooth and of desired consistency.

4. Serve hot, or refrigerate tightly covered for up to 4 days.

PINCH OF SAGE

This gravy is great served hot over fried potatoes or toast. Experiment and see what else you enjoy it over!

Salsas and Relishes

In This Chapter

- Low-sodium accompaniments
- Fresh salsas and relishes
- Flavorful go-withs
- Sneaking in more fruits and veggies

Salsas and relishes can add the perfect zing to an otherwise ho-hum meal. Fish, meats, poultry, egg dishes, snacks, and more can benefit from a well-crafted blend of flavors.

What's more, accompaniments are most often easy to prepare. If you can chop and stir, you can whip up a fresh-tasting, meal-making medley. Nutrient-imparting ingredients; simple preparation; and big, zesty flavor will keep you craving these salsas and relishes.

Singing the Praises of Medleys

You may have been avoiding scooping on salsas or relishes because those jars available in supermarkets contain so much sodium. The good news is that these medleys of tasty vegetables, luscious fruits, and complementary flavorings are often quick, simple recipes to prepare yourself, requiring little more effort than stirring together fresh ingredients.

The vegetables and fruits that make up mouthwatering medleys not only liven up ordinary meals but also add more healthful nutrients to your diet. And effortlessly, to boot!

PINCH OF SAGE

If you prefer ready-made salsas and relishes, some sodium-free, no-salt-added, and low-sodium varieties are available. Check the aisles of your local supermarket.

Relishing Accompaniments

Salsas and relishes can be the hit of your meal. Their fresh tastes and bold flavors make a statement at the table. For an even bigger impact, why not have some fun with your accompaniments? Serve a salsa or relish in a hollowed-out watermelon shell, pineapple rind, zucchini or cucumber boat, avocado peel, orange rind, bell pepper, or any other attractive and sturdy vegetable or fruit shell.

You can serve a salsa or relish at any meal because just about any food you find becomes even tastier with its addition. Fish and seafood, poultry, beef, pork, egg dishes, baked potatoes, and rice are good choices. Give these accompaniments a try on sandwiches, tacos, burritos, and burgers, too. Of course, you can always scoop up a salsa with a tortilla chip (a no-salt-added one, of course). With a little imagination, you'll find many ways to enjoy these salsas and relishes.

Blushing Pear Salsa

Juicy pears are blushed by red onions and flavored by lime and cilantro in this fruit salsa.

Yield:	Prep time:	Chill time:	Serving size:
2¾ cups	15 minutes	8 hours	¼ cup
Each serving has:			
22.1 calories	0.6 mg sodium		

2 medium ripe pears, skin on, cored, and diced

½ cup minced red onions

Juice of 1 lime

2 TB. chopped fresh cilantro

1. In a medium glass bowl, combine pears and red onions. Drizzle lime juice over top, and stir to coat. Stir in cilantro until evenly distributed.

2. Cover and chill overnight. Stir again before serving.

3. Serve with grilled fish or chicken or low-sodium cinnamon pita chips. Refrigerate any leftovers tightly covered for 1 or 2 days.

PINCH OF SAGE

If you don't have time to chill this salsa for several hours, you can serve it after thoroughly chilling for a couple hours. The long chilling time allows for the flavors to mingle, as well as for the red onions to bleed onto the pears, causing the "blushing."

∽

Caribbean Beach Fruit Salsa

Tropical fruits cool the fiery jalapeño and cayenne additions to this fruity salsa.

Yield:	Prep time:	Chill time:	Serving size:
6 cups	20 minutes	1 hour	¼ cup

Each serving has:			
27.7 calories	0.9 mg sodium		

1 (20-oz.) can crushed pineapple, with juice

1½ cups peeled and finely chopped mango

1 cup peeled and finely chopped papaya

1 cup finely diced red onions

½ cup minced fresh jalapeño peppers

Juice of 3 limes

¼ tsp. ground cayenne

1. In a medium bowl, combine pineapple, mango, papaya, red onions, jalapeño peppers, lime juice, and cayenne. Gently stir until blended.

2. Cover and chill for at least 1 hour before serving. Serve alongside grilled or broiled fish, chicken breast, pork, or steak, as desired. Refrigerate any leftovers tightly covered for 2 or 3 days.

PINCH OF SAGE

You can easily remove the seeds from a halved papaya by scooping them out with a metal spoon.

Fresh-Taste Tomato Salsa

Southwestern flavors kick up the taste of garden-picked tomatoes with the added zip of jalapeños.

Yield:	Prep time:	Serving size:
1½ cups	5 minutes	2 tablespoons

Each serving has:		
7.6 calories	1 mg sodium	

1½ cups diced tomatoes (about 2 medium), cored

¼ cup finely diced sweet onions

2 TB. minced jalapeño peppers (about 1 medium), or more to taste

1 tsp. fresh lime juice

1 tsp. dried cilantro or 1 TB. chopped fresh cilantro

1. In a medium bowl, stir together tomatoes, sweet onions, jalapeño peppers, lime juice, and cilantro.

2. If not serving immediately, chill until serving time. Refrigerate any leftovers tightly covered for up to 1 week.

SALT PITFALL

It's worth repeating: wash your hands carefully after cutting the jalapeño pepper (or at least before you rub your eye). The oil that gets on your hands can burn.

Cranberry-Apple Relish

Traditional harvest spices move the classic duo of cranberries and apples from dessert to condiment.

Yield:	Prep time:	Cook time:	Serving size:
3½ cups	5 minutes	25 minutes	¼ cup

Each serving has:			
80 calories	1.3 mg sodium		

1 cup water

¾ cup granulated sugar

1 (12-oz.) pkg. fresh or frozen cranberries

1 cup peeled, diced Braeburn apples (about 1)

½ cup golden raisins

½ cup cider vinegar

¾ tsp. ground cinnamon

½ tsp. ground allspice

¼ tsp. ground cloves

¼ tsp. ground ginger

1. In a medium saucepan over medium heat, combine water and sugar. Bring to a boil, and stir in cranberries, apples, golden raisins, cider vinegar, cinnamon, allspice, cloves, and ginger. Bring to a boil again, and simmer, stirring occasionally, for 10 minutes.

2. Transfer relish into a serving bowl, directly cover surface with plastic wrap, and cool to room temperature.

3. Serve with pork, or cover and chill, bringing relish to room temperature before serving. Refrigerate any leftovers tightly covered for 3 to 5 days.

Salternative: You can substitute your favorite apple in this spicy relish. Try Granny Smith, Golden Delicious, Red Delicious, Gala, Fuji, Jonagold, Pink Lady, or Cameo. You can also adjust the seasonings to taste because it's a very spicy relish.

Flaming Watermelon Salsa

The refreshing taste of watermelon and kiwifruit pairs with the heat of jalapeños for a taste sensation.

Yield:	Prep time:	Serving size:
1½ cups	10 minutes	¼ cup
Each serving has:		
16.4 calories	1.7 mg sodium	

1 cup diced seedless watermelon	2 TB. minced sweet onions
¼ cup peeled, diced kiwifruit	1 TB. balsamic vinegar
3 TB. seeded, minced fresh jalapeño peppers	Pinch garlic powder

1. In a small glass bowl, combine watermelon, kiwifruit, jalapeño peppers, sweet onions, balsamic vinegar, and garlic powder. Stir with a wooden spoon to mix well.

2. Serve with grilled or broiled fish, eggs, cream cheese, or low-sodium crackers. Cover and chill if not serving immediately. Refrigerate any leftovers tightly covered for 1 or 2 days.

Tropical Breeze Pineapple-Orange Salsa

Sweet bites of fruits and bell peppers are flavored by the classic combination of jalapeño, lime, and cilantro.

Yield:	Prep time:	Chill time:	Serving size:
4 cups	15 minutes	1 hour	¼ cup
Each serving has:			
23.7 calories	1.7 mg sodium		

2½ cups bite-size fresh pineapple chunks	2 TB. seeded, minced jalapeño peppers
1 (15-oz.) can mandarin orange segments, drained and halved	1 TB. fresh lime juice
½ cup finely diced red bell pepper	1 tsp. finely chopped fresh cilantro

1. In a large bowl, combine pineapple chunks, mandarin orange segments, red bell pepper, jalapeño peppers, lime juice, and cilantro. Gently stir to mix.

2. Cover and chill for at least 1 hour to allow flavors to blend. Serve with chicken or white fish as desired. Refrigerate any leftovers tightly covered for 1 or 2 days.

PINCH OF SAGE

To remove the crown of a fresh pineapple, twist the crown until it separates from the pineapple. Then you can cut the pineapple in half, cut around and discard the core, slice off the peel, and chop the flesh as needed.

Southwestern Relish

Gussy up your tomato salsa with the Tex-Mex additions of sweet corn and creamy avocado.

Yield:	Prep time:	Serving size:
2 cups	5 minutes	1/3 cup
Each serving has:		
40.4 calories	3.2 mg sodium	

½ cup frozen corn kernels, thawed

½ cup diced avocado

1 cup Fresh-Taste Tomato Salsa (recipe earlier in this chapter)

1. In a medium bowl, stir together corn, avocado, and Fresh-Taste Tomato Salsa.

2. Serve with Fiery Steak with Southwestern Relish (recipe in Chapter 17) or low-sodium tortillas chips. If not serving immediately, chill tightly covered until serving time.

PINCH OF SAGE

To thaw corn kernels quickly, place the corn in a strainer or colander and run it under warm water.

Asian-Flavored Carrot Crunch Salsa

The zing of ginger and jalapeños combine with the crunch of peanuts in this carrot, zucchini, and green onion jumble.

Yield:	Prep time:	Serving size:
6 cups	30 minutes	1/4 cup
Each serving has:		
34.6 calories	6.5 mg sodium	

2½ cups grated carrots

2½ cups grated zucchini

½ cup thinly sliced green onions

⅓ cup unsalted dry-roasted peanuts

2 TB. toasted sesame seeds

1½ medium jalapeño peppers, minced

1 (1-in.) piece fresh gingerroot, peeled and minced

2 TB. extra-virgin olive oil

¼ cup sodium-free rice vinegar

1 tsp. granulated sugar

1. In a large bowl, combine carrots, zucchini, green onions, peanuts, sesame seeds, jalapeño peppers, and gingerroot.

2. In a small bowl, stir together extra-virgin olive oil, rice vinegar, and sugar. Pour over carrot mixture, and stir to coat.

3. Serve with Breakfast Stir-Fry Scramble Pita (recipe in Chapter 3) or low-sodium tortilla chips. Refrigerate any leftovers tightly covered for 3 to 5 days.

Salternative: You can reduce this recipe as needed.

PINCH OF SAGE

You can purchase sesame seeds toasted, but if you want to toast them yourself, heat them in a dry skillet over medium heat for 2 to 5 minutes, shaking occasionally. Cool before using.

Indian Cool Cucumber Raita

This lightly seasoned, creamy blend is traditionally served to cool the palate after eating hot and spicy foods.

Yield:	Prep time:	Chill time:	Serving size:
1¾ cups	20 minutes	2 hours	¼ cup
Each serving has:			
21.9 calories	19.7 mg sodium		

1 medium cucumber, peeled and seeded	1 medium clove garlic, crushed
1 cup fat-free plain yogurt	2 tsp. chopped fresh cilantro
¼ tsp. ground cumin	

1. Grate cucumber into a strainer, and set over the sink to drain.

2. Meanwhile, in a serving bowl, combine yogurt, cumin, and garlic. Stir to blend.

3. Rinse cucumber, and thoroughly press out water. Stir cucumber into yogurt mixture until well blended, and garnish with cilantro.

4. Cover and chill for at least 2 hours or until well chilled and flavors are blended.

PINCH OF SAGE

To seed a cucumber easily, cut in half or into thirds. Then, scoop out the seeds by running a metal spoon between the seeds and the flesh.

Caraway-Beet Relish

Rosy beets are bathed in citrusy orange flavor and studded with the distinctive flavor of caraway seeds.

Yield:	Prep time:	Cook time:	Serving size:
2½ cups	15 minutes	50 minutes	¼ cup

Each serving has:			
43.9 calories	26.6 mg sodium		

5 or 6 medium fresh beets (enough to yield 2 cups, diced)	1 TB. white vinegar
1 small yellow onion, minced	1 TB. unsalted butter
1 rib celery, minced	Zest of 1 orange
3 TB. granulated sugar	Juice of 1 orange
	¼ tsp. caraway seeds

1. Fill a large stainless-steel saucepan with water, and bring to a boil over high heat.

2. Scrub beets and cut off tops, leaving at least 1 inch of stems.

3. Reduce heat to medium, add whole beets to the saucepan, and simmer for 20 to 25 minutes or until beets are fork-tender. Remove beets to a paper towel. Peel with your fingers under cold, running water, and cut off roots and stems. Dice to measure 2 cups.

4. Rinse out the saucepan, and add 2 cups diced beets, onion, celery, sugar, white vinegar, butter, orange zest, orange juice, and caraway seeds. Stir. Bring to a simmer over medium heat, reduce heat to medium-low, and simmer for 20 minutes. Cool.

5. Cover tightly, and chill in a glass bowl for up to 1 month. Serve with pork or beef, as desired.

SALT PITFALL

Staining is a concern when cooking beets. Wash all surfaces immediately if splatters occur. Don't use a wooden cutting board or a wooden spoon because they'll be purple when you're done! Instead, opt for materials that won't permanently stain.

Slathers, Spreads, and Seasoning Blends

In This Chapter

- Flavoring without salt
- Spreading great taste with savory butters
- Sweetening each bite with fruit butters
- Shaking on salt-free seasonings

You, your family, and your guests all warmly welcome flavorful foods. Salt has been the greatest flavor enhancer throughout history, and if you're finding yourself without a good salt-alternative seasoning, don't despair. You can infuse flavor with just a little slather, spread, or seasoning blend.

Even better, butters and seasonings are easy to make. With just a little effort, you can whip up rich, complex flavors that will make you wonder why you were ever so dependent on your salt shaker.

Wait 'Til You Smear!

Butters, both sweet and savory, are tasty additions to breads, rolls, buns, biscuits, quick breads, muffins, pancakes, waffles, French toast, and more. A once-plain food can take on new appeal when the smear is delicious.

Any leftover savory butters are perfect for seasoning cooked vegetables. Perk up green beans, corn, baked potatoes, carrots, mushrooms, and more.

Shake It Up, Baby

Because you've put away the salt shaker, you may need to mix up your own seasoning blends to spice up your favorite foods. Several commercially prepared seasoning mixes often include salt or even MSG as an ingredient. The recipes in this chapter should help you substitute for those blends most difficult to find without added salt.

Many seasoning blends are available without salt, though. Check your local supermarket's spice aisle, or find a mail-order supplier of salt-free seasonings. Even though the spice aisle is teeming with salt-free salt substitute seasoning blends in a wide variety of mixes, we've included a recipe here in case you want to mix up your own.

> **SALT PITFALL**
>
> When picking up seasoning blends from your supermarket's spice aisle, always read the labels carefully. Vigilantly check such seasoning mixes as chili powder, curry powder, garlic-pepper blend, lemon-pepper, poultry seasoning, seafood seasoning, salad seasoning, and any of the specialty seasoning blends. Often, salt is the primary ingredient.

Making your own seasoning blends is an inexpensive alternative to the store-bought versions. Plus, if you have 5 minutes, you can create a flavor-imparting seasoning blend.

Fast Fish Seasoning Blend

A mix of herbs keeps this salt-free blend light and fresh.

Yield:	Prep time:	Serving size:
10 teaspoons	5 minutes	¼ teaspoon
Each serving has:		
0.9 calories	0.2 mg sodium	

1 TB. dried thyme	½ tsp. garlic powder
1 TB. dried chives	½ tsp. dried lemon peel
½ TB. dried basil	¼ tsp. dried mint
1 tsp. dried parsley flakes	⅛ tsp. ground cayenne

1. In a small, airtight spice jar, combine thyme, chives, basil, parsley flakes, garlic powder, lemon peel, mint, and cayenne. Cover and shake well to combine.

2. Store in a cool, dry place for up to 6 months.

PINCH OF SAGE

This seasoning blend is pretty versatile. Combine ⅛ teaspoon with melted butter or oil, and brush over a 3-ounce fish fillet. You also can use it dry, if you prefer to cut the fat. Try it on chicken or pasta as well.

Sweet Strawberry Butter

Sugar-sweetened strawberries make this buttery spread delectable.

Yield:	Prep time:	Chill time:	Serving size:
2¼ cups	5 minutes	3 hours	2 tablespoons
Each serving has:			
109.4 calories	0.2 mg sodium		

1½ cups fresh strawberries, rinsed, hulled, and quartered

¾ cup (1½ sticks) unsalted butter, softened

1½ cups confectioners' sugar

1. In a blender, combine strawberries, butter, and confectioners' sugar. Blend on high speed for 1 or 2 minutes or until thoroughly blended, scraping down the sides as necessary.

2. Pour strawberry butter into a storage container with a tight-fitting lid. Chill for at least 3 hours to firm up a bit. Store in the refrigerator tightly covered for up to 1 week.

Salternative: You can decrease this recipe as needed.

PINCH OF SAGE

Spread this scrumptious butter over your morning pancakes or waffles, and try it on biscuits or slices of sweet breads.

Herb-Flecked Butter

Fresh herbs add their bright taste to this buttery spread.

Yield:	Prep time:	Chill time:	Serving size:
¼ cup	10 minutes	8 hours	1 teaspoon
Each serving has:			
33.6 calories	0.3 mg sodium		

4 TB. unsalted butter, cut into small pieces and softened	1 tsp. chopped fresh basil
1½ TB. chopped fresh parsley	¾ tsp. chopped fresh tarragon

1. In a small bowl, combine butter, parsley, basil, and tarragon. Stir until herbs are evenly distributed.

2. Spoon mixture onto a small sheet of waxed paper. Shape into a log, and wrap in the waxed paper. Chill overnight until firm and flavors are blended.

3. Store in the refrigerator tightly wrapped for up to 1 week.

Salt-Shaker Substitute

This salt substitute gives your recipes a spicy flair. Fill your salt shaker with it, and get used to shaking it on foods you like salt on.

Yield:	Prep time:	Serving size:
2½ tablespoons	5 minutes	¼ teaspoon
Each serving has:		
2.1 calories	0.3 mg sodium	

1 TB. onion powder	½ tsp. paprika
1½ tsp. ground dry mustard	½ tsp. Firehouse Chili Powder (recipe later in this chapter) or other salt-free chili powder
1½ tsp. dried basil	
½ tsp. celery seeds	

1. In a small, airtight spice jar, combine onion powder, dry mustard, basil, celery seeds, paprika, and Firehouse Chili Powder. Cover and shake well to combine.

2. Store in a cool, dry place for up to 6 months.

Festive Green Pistachio Butter

Smooth, blanched pistachios speckle this spring- or holiday-colored buttery spread.

Yield:	Prep time:	Cook time:	Serving size:
1/3 cup	15 minutes	5 minutes	1 teaspoon
Each serving has:			
47.8 calories	0.4 mg sodium		

1/2 cup unsalted unshelled natural pistachios

4 TB. unsalted butter, melted

2 drops green food coloring (optional)

1. Fill a small saucepan with water, and bring to a boil over high heat. Add pistachios, and remove from heat. Let stand for 1 or 2 minutes and then drain. Shell pistachios and peel off papery covering.

2. Place pistachios in a zipper-lock bag, and pound with a rolling pin or a meat mallet until pistachios reach a fine to medium crumble.

3. In a small bowl, blend together butter and pistachios with a spoon until evenly distributed. Add food coloring (if using), and stir until evenly colored.

4. Pack butter into a serving crock. Cover tightly and chill for up to 1 week, softening slightly before serving.

Salternative: You can decrease or increase this recipe as needed.

PINCH OF SAGE

Some pistachios are still sold coated in their familiar bright red dye. The dye was once added because manufacturers wanted to mask the natural imperfections that mar the nuts' appearance. Because you'll be plunging these pistachios into boiling water, you can't substitute the red-dyed pistachios for the natural nuts.

Lemon-Bright Cilantro Butter

This buttery spread heightens the flavor of cilantro with a splash of lemon juice.

Yield:	Prep time:	Chill time:	Serving size:
¼ cup	10 minutes	1 hour	1 teaspoon
Each serving has:			
33.8 calories	0.7 mg sodium		

4 TB. unsalted butter, softened

¼ cup finely chopped fresh cilantro

½ tsp. fresh lemon juice

1. In a small bowl, cream together butter and cilantro until well blended. Stir in lemon juice.

2. Spoon mixture onto a small sheet of waxed paper. Shape into a log, and wrap in the waxed paper. Chill for 1 hour or until firm.

3. Soften slightly to slice and serve. Store in the refrigerator tightly wrapped for up to 1 week.

Jerk Seasoning Blend

A heady mix, the heat of this seasoning blend is complemented by classic harvest baking spices.

Yield:	Prep time:	Serving size:
2 tablespoons	2 minutes	1 teaspoon
Each serving has:		
6 calories	12 mg sodium	

1 TB. onion powder

1 tsp. ground allspice

½ tsp. freshly ground black pepper

¼ tsp. cayenne

¼ tsp. ground *chipotle chili pepper*

¼ tsp. garlic powder

¼ tsp. ground cinnamon

¼ tsp. ground nutmeg

⅛ tsp. ground cloves

⅛ tsp. dried thyme

1. In a small, airtight spice jar, combine onion powder, allspice, pepper, cayenne, chipotle chili pepper, garlic powder, cinnamon, nutmeg, cloves, and thyme. Cover and shake well to combine.

2. Store in a cool, dry place for up to 6 months.

Salternative: If you enjoy high heat, substitute ½ teaspoon ground habañero chili pepper for the cayenne and ground chipotle chili pepper called for here.

DEFINITION

Chipotle chili peppers are dried, smoked jalapeño peppers that lend a smoky flavor to recipes.

Overnight Spiced Pumpkin Butter

A concentration of fall flavors adds a punch of pumpkin to your meals.

Yield:	Prep time:	Cook time:	Serving size:
3⅔ cups	5 minutes	13 hours	2 tablespoons
Each serving has:			
56 calories	1.6 mg sodium		

1 (29-oz.) can solid-packed pumpkin (not pumpkin pie filling)	1¾ cups granulated sugar 1 tsp. pumpkin pie spice

1. In a 2- or 3-quart slow cooker, combine pumpkin, sugar, and pumpkin pie spice. Stir to blend. Cover and cook on high for 1 hour.

2. Reduce temperature to low, and continue to cook for 12 hours.

3. Cool and store tightly covered in the refrigerator for up to 2 weeks. Spread on toast, bagels, crackers, muffins, quick breads, pancakes, or waffles, or stir into oatmeal or yogurt, as desired.

Southern Heat BBQ Dry Rub

Heat with just a touch of sweet will rub your taste buds the right way.

Yield:	Prep time:	Serving size:
9 tablespoons	5 minutes	½ tablespoon

Each serving has:		
18 calories	2 mg sodium	

3 TB. *paprika*

3 TB. firmly packed dark brown sugar

1 TB. Firehouse Chili Powder (recipe later in this chapter) or other salt-free chili powder

2 tsp. freshly ground black pepper

1 tsp. cayenne

1 tsp. ground cumin

1 tsp. garlic powder

1 tsp. onion powder

1. In a small, airtight spice jar, combine paprika, dark brown sugar, Firehouse Chili Powder, pepper, cayenne, cumin, garlic powder, and onion powder. Cover and shake well to combine.

2. Store in a cool, dry place for up to 6 months.

DEFINITION

Paprika is a spice ground from dried red peppers. Blends marked as simply "paprika" tend to be sweeter blends. Heat lovers may prefer the hot paprika versions.

Asian-Inspired Spice Blend

This mix combines heat with undertones of anise and cloves.

Yield:	Prep time:	Serving size:
5 tablespoons	5 minutes	1 teaspoon
Each serving has:		
7 calories	3 mg sodium	

2 TB. ground ginger

2 TB. crushed red pepper flakes

2 tsp. ground black pepper

2 tsp. anise seeds

1½ tsp. ground cloves

1 tsp. ground white pepper

1. In a small, airtight spice jar, combine ginger, crushed red pepper flakes, pepper, anise seeds, cloves, and white pepper. Cover and shake well to combine.

2. Store in a cool, dry place for up to 6 months.

Salternative: If you don't care for the heat of this mix, reduce the crushed red pepper flakes as desired. You can adjust all premixed seasonings to taste.

PINCH OF SAGE

Sprinkle this blend dry into stir-fries or rice dishes, or mix with a little sesame oil. You may also try it on Grilled Asian-Spiced Chicken Thighs (recipe in Chapter 16).

Taco Seasoning Mix

This salt-free seasoning mix adds Mexican flavors, thanks to the heat-providing spices.

Yield:	Prep time:	Serving size:
1½ teaspoons	5 minutes	1½ teaspoons
Each serving has:		
11.4 calories	3.2 mg sodium	

½ tsp. Firehouse Chili Powder
   (recipe later in this chapter) or
   other salt-free chili powder
¼ tsp. freshly ground black pepper

¼ tsp. ground cumin
¼ tsp. dried oregano
¼ tsp. ground cayenne

1. In a small, airtight spice jar, combine Firehouse Chili Powder, pepper, cumin, oregano, and cayenne. Cover and shake well to combine.

2. Store in a cool, dry place for up to 6 months.

Salternative: The Firehouse Chili Powder is a bit on the hot side. You can substitute a commercially prepared salt-free spice blend if you want.

PINCH OF SAGE

This recipe makes enough seasoning mix to flavor 1 pound meat. Increase this recipe to keep a spice jar available for quick use.

Firehouse Chili Powder

Smoking hot, this salt-free chili powder adds heat when needed.

Yield:	Prep time:	Serving size:
5 tablespoons	10 minutes	1 teaspoon

Each serving has:		
10.6 calories	3.5 mg sodium	

⅓ cup crushed red pepper flakes

4 tsp. ground cumin

2 tsp. garlic powder

1 tsp. dried oregano

1 tsp. ground chipotle chili pepper

1. In a mini food chopper or a food processor, combine crushed red pepper flakes, cumin, garlic powder, oregano, and chipotle chili pepper. Process for 2 or 3 minutes or until well combined and powdered.

2. Store in an airtight spice jar or other container in a cool, dry place for up to 6 months.

SALT PITFALL

When shopping for chili powder, even if the label doesn't disclose salt, look for other sodium keywords, such as *monosodium glutamate,* or *MSG. Spices* or *natural seasonings* may be listed as an ingredient as well. You can contact the manufacturer to find out if the product includes salt or another sodium product.

Marvelous Main Dishes

Perhaps the most repeated question, day in and day out, is "What's for dinner?" If you're new to cooking without salt or added sodium, you may dread the daily question. But you don't have to. The recipes in Part 5 give you a selection of dishes with a variety of ingredients encompassing a range of cooking times. Whether you need a fast-fix family meal or a dinner-party entrée, you'll find a recipe to prepare and savor.

Fish and seafood, poultry, beef, pork, and meatless main dishes give you the meals necessary to please your pickiest eaters, vary your dinnertime options, and keep your sodium intake at responsible levels. Moreover, the diversity of main dishes allows you to take advantage of each meal's nutrients and other health benefits. But most of your partakers will only care about the great taste. Ring the dinner bell, and watch them dig in!

Fish and Seafood Entrées

In This Chapter

- Purchasing fresh fish and seafood
- Cooking quick and nutritious meals
- Including omega-3 essential fatty acids in your diet
- Limiting certain fish

Fish and seafood are perfect for busy families because a meal from the ocean cooks up quickly. Plus, fish and seafood can carry a wide array of seasonings and flavors, so your family is sure to find a dish to savor.

You'll feel good, too, knowing you're serving your family a healthful dinner. Shellfish provide a lean protein that's low in fat and carbohydrates. The fat in oily, cold-water fish like salmon serves up a healthful dose of omega-3 essential fatty acids. With all that going for you, what are you waiting for? Pick a recipe, and let's get cooking!

Buying the Best Catch

For the best flavor and convenience, purchase fresh fish and seafood that's properly iced or refrigerated. If you buy only from a reputable vendor, you're unlikely to see fish with a brown or yellowish discoloration or darkening around the edges—clues the fish isn't fresh. The flesh of a fresh fish should spring back when you press it. Don't buy fish that's soft or mushy. Finally, fresh fish and seafood smell mild and fresh with almost no odor. A fishy smell points to decomposition.

To maintain the freshness of your fish and seafood purchases, refrigerate or freeze your selections immediately when you get home. If you live any distance from the supermarket or fish market, if the weather is warm, or if you'll be storing your groceries in a hot car trunk, take along a cooler to pack your cold-storage food items in. Just be sure to separate your fish, poultry, and meats from each other and your other foods—just as you did in your shopping cart.

Cook fresh fish and seafood within a day or two. If you won't be using it in that time span, place it in the freezer, properly packaged against freezer burn. Airtight packages of heavy aluminum foil, plastic freezer wrap, and zipper-lock freezer bags will keep your fish and seafood protected for 4 to 6 months in the freezer.

Fish that was previously frozen must be identified at the supermarket or fish market. Plan on cooking any such purchases in a day or two because they should not be refrozen.

Preparation Pointers

When you prepare fish and seafood, remember to follow safe-handling rules. Use separate utensils, dishes, and cutting boards for raw fish and seafood. Wash your hands in warm, soapy water before and after handling it. Thaw frozen fish and seafood in the refrigerator overnight. If you're in a pinch, you can thaw it in the microwave just until it's icy and malleable, but be sure to cook it immediately.

Fish and seafood are great choices for fast meals because they typically cook in just 5 to 20 minutes. When baking or broiling, plan on cooking for a total of 10 minutes per inch of thickness. You can tell fish and seafood are thoroughly cooked when the flesh turns opaque. Fin fish will also flake easily with a fork.

SALT PITFALL

Overcooking fish and seafood results in a rubbery, chewy texture, so be sure to stop cooking as soon as it's opaque.

Fishing for Good Health

Oily, cold-water fish such as salmon, lake trout, tuna, herring, sardines, and mackerel contain omega-3 *essential fatty acids*. Because your body cannot make this type of poly-unsaturated fat itself, you need to get it from food sources to reap the benefits. Research indicates that omega-3 fatty acids may promote heart health, protect against some cancers, ease depression, and facilitate improvement of some autoimmune disorders.

DEFINITION

Essential fatty acids are a type of polyunsaturated fat your body gets from foods. Your body is not able to make such fatty acids itself.

With the high praises of fish as a nutritional boon come the cautions of contamination. Some fish have been found to contain high levels of mercury. Therefore, it's recommended you limit swordfish, shark, king mackerel, and tilefish to just one serving a month (for healthy adults). Check with your local extension office for up-to-date advisories as well as local fish-eating guidelines.

Hot and Sweet Mustard–Crusted Salmon

The zippy sauce topping this salmon fillet is cut with an undertone of sweetness.

Yield:	Prep time:	Cook time:	Serving size:
4 servings	5 minutes	11 minutes	4 ounces fish
Each serving has:			
247.2 calories	58.1 mg sodium		

1 lb. skin-on salmon

1 TB. dry mustard

1 TB. granulated sugar

1 tsp. water

¼ tsp. dried dill weed

1. Preheat the broiler to high. Spray the rack of a broiler pan with nonstick cooking spray.

2. Place salmon skin side down on the rack. Broil 4 to 6 inches from heat for 10 minutes per inch of thickness or until salmon flakes easily with a fork.

3. Meanwhile, in a small bowl, combine dry mustard, sugar, and water. Stir until thick paste forms and then stir in dill weed. Spread mixture evenly over top of salmon.

4. Return to broiler, and broil for 1 minute or until browned and bubbly.

PINCH OF SAGE

To serve skin-on salmon, cut through the salmon down to, but not through, the skin for each serving. Slide a spatula between the skin and the flesh to remove each piece.

Lemon-Paprika Grouper

A lightly seasoned lemon-butter sauce coats fillets of tasty whitefish.

Yield:	Prep time:	Cook time:	Serving size:
4 servings	10 minutes	12 minutes	4 ounces fish

Each serving has:	
157.5 calories	61.7 mg sodium

2 TB. unsalted butter, melted	1/4 tsp. ground white pepper
1/2 TB. fresh lemon juice	1/4 tsp. paprika
1/2 tsp. dried parsley flakes	1 lb. grouper fillets
1/4 tsp. garlic powder	

1. Preheat the oven to 350°F. Position the oven rack in the upper-middle position. Cover the rack of a broiler pan with aluminum foil.

2. In a small bowl, combine butter and lemon juice. Brush about 1/2 tablespoon lemon-butter mixture onto the foil where fillets will be.

3. In another small bowl, combine parsley flakes, garlic powder, white pepper, and paprika. Sprinkle 1/2 of mixture on undersides of fillets. Place fillets, seasoning side down, on the prepared foil. Sprinkle remaining seasoning mixture over top of fillets.

4. Bake for 12 minutes or until fish flakes easily with a fork. Brush remaining butter mixture over fillets.

PINCH OF SAGE

Be sure to cover the broiler rack completely with aluminum foil, shaping it to the pan. Then you can just toss the foil—no pan scrubbing!

Veggie-Lover's Crunchy Tuna Noodle Casserole

The classic creamy baked dish is packed with colorful vegetables topped off with a tortilla chip crunch.

Yield:	Prep time:	Cook time:	Serving size:
6 cups	25 minutes	15 minutes	1½ cups

Each serving has:			
361 calories	67.1 mg sodium		

4 cups uncooked wide egg noodles

2 TB. unsalted butter

1 small yellow onion, diced

1 medium clove garlic, minced

¼ cup diced red bell pepper

¼ cup diced green bell pepper

¼ cup diced carrots

1 TB. all-purpose flour

1 cup fat-free milk

1 tsp. Salt-Shaker Substitute (recipe in Chapter 14) or other salt-free salt substitute seasoning blend

¼ tsp. freshly ground black pepper

½ cup drained no-salt-added canned peas

1 (6-oz.) can very low-sodium albacore tuna packed in water, drained and flaked

½ cup crushed unsalted tortilla chips

1. Preheat the oven to 350°F. Spray a 1½-quart glassware casserole dish with nonstick cooking spray.

2. Cook egg noodles according to the package directions (omit salt). Drain.

3. Meanwhile, in a large nonstick skillet over medium heat, melt 1 tablespoon butter. Add onion, garlic, red bell pepper, green bell pepper, and carrots, and sauté for 5 minutes or until softened.

4. In a small saucepan over medium heat, melt remaining 1 tablespoon butter. Whisk in flour, and when smooth and bubbly, gradually whisk in milk. Bring to a simmer, and whisk for 1 or 2 minutes or until slightly thickened. Turn off heat.

5. Stir in Salt-Shaker Substitute and pepper. Add onion mixture, and stir in peas, tuna, and egg noodles until combined.

6. Place mixture in the prepared casserole dish, and sprinkle tortilla chip crumbs on top. Bake for 15 to 20 minutes or until browned and heated through.

PINCH OF SAGE

An easy way to crush the tortilla chips—and take out any frustration you might be feeling—is to close the chips in a zipper-lock bag and pound them with the flat side of a meat mallet or a rolling pin.

Lemon Cod Pockets

This dill-seasoned whitefish is steamed with sweet red peppers and mild green onions.

Yield:	Prep time:	Cook time:	Serving size:
4 servings	15 minutes	10 minutes	1 pocket
Each serving has:			
129.9 calories	75.3 mg sodium		

4 tsp. unsalted butter

4 (4-oz.) cod loin fillets

¼ tsp. freshly ground black pepper

1 medium lemon, sliced and seeded

1 medium red bell pepper, ribs and seeds removed, and thinly sliced

4 medium green onions, trimmed and coarsely chopped

1 tsp. dried dill weed

1. Preheat the oven to 400°F.

2. Place 1 teaspoon butter in the center of each of 4 large sheets of nonstick aluminum foil. Place 1 cod fillet on top of butter. Season fillets with pepper, and lay lemon slices atop each. Scatter red bell pepper and green onions over top, and season all with dill weed. Close foil pockets, double-sealing the seams.

3. Bake for 10 to 12 minutes or until fish flakes easily with a fork.

PINCH OF SAGE

Make up these pockets in the morning or even the night before to have ready to pop into the oven for a quick-fix dinner.

Mahimahi Stir-Fry

With a splash of sesame seed oil and soy sauce substitute, fresh ginger and classic Chinese flavors surround these meaty whitefish pieces.

Yield:	Prep time:	Cook time:	Serving size:
5 cups	3 minutes	13 minutes	1¼ cups
Each serving has:			
206.2 calories	115.9 mg sodium		

3 tsp. canola oil

3 TB. cornstarch

12 oz. mahimahi, fresh or thawed frozen, and cut into 2-in. cubes

1 cup (1-in.) lengths asparagus spears

1 cup julienned carrots

1 cup halved and thinly sliced yellow onions

1 cup julienned red bell peppers

1 cup sliced button mushrooms

2 medium cloves garlic, minced

1½ TB. peeled and grated fresh gingerroot

½ tsp. crushed red pepper flakes

1 tsp. sesame seed oil

¼ cup Sodium-Wise Soy Sauce Stand-In (recipe in Chapter 12)

1. Heat a wok or very large skillet over medium-high heat. Add 2 teaspoons canola oil.

2. Place cornstarch in a small, shallow bowl.

3. Dredge mahimahi in cornstarch, shaking off any excess. Add to the wok, and stir-fry for 3 minutes or until fish is opaque. Using a slotted spoon, transfer mahimahi to a plate.

4. Add remaining 1 teaspoon canola oil to the wok. Add asparagus, carrots, onions, and red bell peppers, and stir-fry for 3 minutes.

5. Add mushrooms, garlic, gingerroot, crushed red pepper flakes, and sesame seed oil, and stir-fry for 5 minutes or until vegetables are crisp-tender.

6. Stir in Sodium-Wise Soy Sauce Stand-In, and return mahimahi to the wok. Stir-fry for 2 minutes or until heated through and evenly coated. Serve over cooked brown rice or lo mein noodles, as desired.

PINCH OF SAGE

When working with fresh gingerroot, you've got to peel it first. That's easy, using a vegetable peeler.

Tilapia Florentine

A creamy spinach sauce flavors this mild whitefish.

Yield:	Prep time:	Cook time:	Serving size:
4 servings	15 minutes	20 minutes	1 casserole
Each serving has:			
179.5 calories	128 mg sodium		

2 TB. extra-virgin olive oil	4 (3.5-oz.) tilapia fillets, rinsed and patted dry with paper towels
4 cups packed, washed and stemmed spinach leaves	1 TB. all-purpose flour
2 medium green onions, trimmed and thinly sliced	1 cup fat-free milk
½ tsp. dried marjoram	⅛ tsp. freshly ground black pepper
1 TB. grated lemon zest	1 medium lemon, thinly sliced

1. Preheat the oven to 400°F. Spray 4 individual glassware casserole dishes with non-stick cooking spray.

2. In a large skillet over medium heat, heat extra-virgin olive oil. Add spinach and green onions, and sauté for 3 minutes or until spinach is wilted.

3. Divide spinach mixture among the prepared casserole dishes, and sprinkle with marjoram and lemon zest. Place tilapia fillets on top.

4. In a small bowl, stir flour into ¼ cup milk.

5. In a small saucepan over medium heat, heat remaining ¾ cup milk, and stir in flour-milk mixture. Cook, stirring, for 3 minutes or until thickened. Stir in pepper, and pour milk sauce over fillets.

6. Arrange lemon slices over fillets, and bake for 20 minutes or until lightly browned and bubbly.

PINCH OF SAGE

These single-serving casseroles make a nice presentation for guests. If you don't have individual casserole dishes, bake this recipe in a 8×8×2-inch or 9×9×2-inch baking dish, alternating head-to-tail placement to fit.

Florentine Tuna-Stuffed Manicotti Casserole

Topped with a spicy cream sauce and juicy tomatoes, these manicotti pasta shells hold a medley of herbed spinach, tuna, and cheese.

Yield:	Prep time:	Cook time:	Serving size:
1 dozen manicotti	25 minutes	45 minutes	2 manicotti

Each serving has:			
420.5 calories	137.3 mg sodium		

2 TB. extra-virgin olive oil

1 cup diced yellow onions

$\frac{1}{8}$ tsp. crushed red pepper flakes (optional)

2 medium cloves garlic, minced

6 cups baby spinach leaves, rinsed and lightly packed

2 (4.5-oz.) cans very-low-sodium albacore tuna, drained

2 tsp. lemon juice

4 TB. chopped fresh Italian parsley

2 TB. chopped fresh basil

3 tsp. Salt-Shaker Substitute (recipe in Chapter 14) or other salt-free salt substitute seasoning blend

12 manicotti pasta shells

2 TB. unsalted butter

2 TB. all-purpose flour

1 cup fat-free milk

$\frac{1}{2}$ tsp. freshly ground black pepper

$1\frac{1}{2}$ cups low-sodium Swiss cheese

1 cup finely diced tomatoes

1. Heat a large skillet over medium to medium-low heat. When hot, add extra-virgin olive oil, and heat for 1 minute. Add onions and crushed red pepper flakes (if using), and cook, stirring occasionally, for 6 minutes or until onions are softened.

2. Add garlic, and cook, stirring, for 1 minute. Add spinach, and cook for 3 minutes or until wilted, stirring occasionally.

3. Stir in tuna, breaking up, and cook for 1 minute or until heated through. Turn off heat.

4. Add lemon juice, 2 tablespoons Italian parsley, basil, and 1 teaspoon Salt-Shaker Substitute, and stir to combine. Set aside.

5. Cook manicotti shells according to package directions (omit salt) until al dente. Drain.

6. Preheat the oven to 350°F. Coat a 13×9×2 casserole dish with nonstick cooking spray.

7. Meanwhile, in a small saucepan over medium heat, melt butter. Whisk in flour until smooth and bubbly. Whisk in milk until smooth. Whisk in remaining 2 teaspoons Salt-Shaker Substitute and pepper until smooth and bubbly. Turn off heat and whisk in remaining 2 tablespoons Italian parsley. Set aside.

8. Lightly cover the bottom of the dish with sauce mixture.

9. Stir Swiss cheese into tuna mixture, and using a small spoon, stuff tuna mixture evenly into manicotti shells (keeping filling enclosed) and arrange in the prepared dish. Spoon sauce over manicotti, covering all evenly, and sprinkle tomatoes over top. Cover and bake for 25 minutes or until hot.

> **PINCH OF SAGE**
>
> Lightly covering the bottom of a casserole dish with a sauce, if the recipe calls for one, helps to prevent sticking and overcooking on the bottom.

Skillet-Sizzled Sea Scallops

The fresh seafood flavor of the scallops shines with a hint of simple seasonings.

Yield:	Prep time:	Cook time:	Serving size:
4 servings	5 minutes	7 minutes	4 ounces scallops

Each serving has:		
231.3 calories	185.2 mg sodium	

5 TB. unsalted butter	Juice of ½ lemon
1 lb. sea scallops, rinsed and patted dry with paper towels	2 tsp. chopped fresh parsley
2 medium cloves garlic, minced	¼ tsp. paprika

1. In a large, nonstick skillet over medium to medium-low heat, melt butter. Add sea scallops and garlic, and cook for 4 or 5 minutes without moving scallops. Turn scallops over, drizzle lemon juice over top, and cook for 3 or 4 minutes or until just opaque.

2. Remove scallops to a serving platter, and sprinkle parsley and paprika over top.

PINCH OF SAGE

When shopping for sea scallops, choose ones that are ivory-colored or a pink-hued beige. Bright white scallops have been processed to extend their shelf life. Avoid these because you won't be able to brown them.

Chinese-Style Shrimp Pasta Primavera

With a touch of ginger and heat, tender-crisp veggies enliven this quick shrimp dish.

Yield:	Prep time:	Cook time:	Serving size:
4 servings	15 minutes	15 minutes	2 ounces pasta with 1 cup shrimp-vegetable mixture

Each serving has:	
429.8 calories	189.5 mg sodium

8 oz. mini penne or other medium pasta

2 TB. extra-virgin olive oil

1 medium yellow onion, cut into thin wedges

3 medium cloves garlic, minced

½ cup *julienned* carrots

½ cup trimmed Chinese snow peas, sliced diagonally if large

1 medium red bell pepper, ribs and seeds removed, and cut into thin strips

2 TB. lemon juice

1 TB. peeled and grated fresh gingerroot

⅛ tsp. crushed red pepper flakes

3 TB. cornstarch

1 (14.5-oz.) can light-sodium fat-free chicken broth

12 oz. medium shrimp (about 34), peeled, and deveined, cooked or uncooked

1. Cook pasta according to the package directions (omit salt). Drain.

2. In a 2-quart microwave-safe casserole dish, combine extra-virgin olive oil, onion, garlic, carrots, snow peas, red bell pepper, lemon juice, gingerroot, and crushed red pepper flakes. Cover, venting, and cook on high for 3 minutes or until vegetables are tender-crisp, stirring halfway through the cooking time.

3. Meanwhile, in a small bowl, whisk cornstarch into chicken broth. Stir into vegetable mixture. Cover, venting, and cook on high for 4 or 5 minutes or until sauce is a little thickened, stirring halfway through the cooking time.

4. Stir in shrimp. Cover, venting, and cook on high for 1½ to 2 minutes or until heated through, stirring halfway through the cooking time.

5. Let stand for 2 minutes before serving over pasta.

> **DEFINITION**
>
> **Julienned** vegetables are sliced into thin, matchsticklike pieces.

Italian Shrimp Fettuccini

Shrimp broth infuses flavor into the basil-tinged tomato and spinach pasta sauce.

Yield:	Prep time:	Cook time:	Serving size:
6 servings	5 minutes	25 minutes	2 ounces pasta with 1 cup sauce

Each serving has:	
363.8 calories	206.5 mg sodium

12 oz. fettuccini	¼ cup fresh lemon juice
1 lb. medium shrimp (about 45), peeled, deveined, and cooked	4 medium cloves garlic, minced
	1 tsp. dried basil
½ cup water	¼ tsp. freshly ground black pepper
1 (10-oz.) pkg. frozen chopped spinach	1 (14.5-oz.) can no-salt-added diced tomatoes, with juice
2 TB. plus 1 tsp. extra-virgin olive oil	

1. Cook fettuccini according to the package directions (omit salt). Drain.

2. Finely chop 2 shrimp, and add to a small microwave-safe bowl with water. Cook, uncovered, on high for 1 minute to make a broth.

3. Unwrap frozen spinach. Place the package on a microwave-safe plate, and cook on high for 3 minutes.

4. Meanwhile, in a medium bowl, combine remaining shrimp, 2 tablespoons extra-virgin olive oil, lemon juice, garlic, basil, and pepper.

5. In a large nonstick skillet over medium heat, heat remaining 1 teaspoon extra-virgin olive oil. Add spinach, tomatoes, and shrimp broth. Increase heat to high, and cook, stirring, for 2 minutes or until boiling.

6. Add shrimp mixture, and cook for 2 minutes or until heated through.

7. To serve, line plates with fettuccini and spoon shrimp and sauce over top.

PINCH OF SAGE

Try to find fresh cooked shrimp, or purchase fresh shrimp and cook it yourself. You can use frozen cooked shrimp, but salt is added to frozen shrimp during processing.

Broiled Salmon with Cherry Tomato Couscous

A warm, lemony vinaigrette flavors whole-wheat pasta with bites of garden-fresh tomatoes in this scrumptious salmon dish.

Yield:	Prep time:	Cook time:	Serving size:
4 servings	5 minutes	15 minutes	3 ounces salmon with 1 heaping cup couscous mixture

Each serving has:	
395.5 calories	304.2 mg sodium

1 (14.5-oz.) can reduced-sodium, fat-free chicken broth

1⅓ cups whole-wheat pearl couscous

2 TB. extra-virgin olive oil

2 TB. lemon juice

⅛ tsp. freshly ground black pepper

2 medium green onions, finely chopped

3 TB. chopped fresh parsley

2 cups halved cherry tomatoes

1 lb. wild salmon fillet

¼ tsp. ground cumin

¼ tsp. garlic powder

1. Preheat the broiler to high. Spray the rack of a broiler pan with nonstick cooking spray.

2. In a small saucepan over high heat, bring chicken broth to a boil. Stir in pearl couscous, and return to a boil. Reduce heat to low, cover, and simmer for 10 to 12 minutes or until broth is absorbed. Fluff couscous with a fork.

3. Meanwhile, in a medium bowl, whisk together extra-virgin olive oil, lemon juice, and pepper. Add couscous, green onions, parsley, and cherry tomatoes, and stir to coat evenly.

4. Place salmon on the rack of the broiler pan skin side down, and season with cumin and garlic powder. Broil 4 to 6 inches from the heat source for 10 minutes for each inch of thickness or until done.

5. To serve, spoon couscous mixture onto serving plates. With a fine, sharp knife, separate salmon flesh from skin and cut into even portions. Arrange salmon atop couscous mixture.

PINCH OF SAGE

You can reduce your sodium intake by replacing reduced-sodium chicken broth called for in a recipe with an equal amount of prepared sodium-free chicken bouillon granules. Sodium-free chicken bouillon granules are made with potassium chloride, so check with your doctor or nutritionist to see if this substitution is right for you.

Pleasing Poultry Dishes

In This Chapter

- Amazingly adaptable poultry
- Making healthful poultry choices
- The importance of safe food handling
- Tasty and diverse chicken and turkey dishes

Poultry is a favorite, thanks to its tender, juicy, meaty portions your whole family will welcome—even the pickiest eaters! Plus, its ease of preparation, as well as the variations it allows (baking, broiling, grilling, roasting, sautéing, oven-frying, and so on) make it a kitchen favorite.

Chicken and turkey offer a mild flavor that acts as a blank canvas for seasonings and other flavors and works equally well with savory or sweet. Even if you serve poultry frequently, you'll find a wide array of seasonings and cooking methods to keep your appetite piqued. Plus poultry's a snap to prepare with as little sodium as possible.

Get ready to shake the old salt-and-pepper routine! The recipes in this chapter take you on a flavorful poultry adventure.

All Parts Are Not Created Equal

Wings, thighs, drumsticks, breasts, tenderloins, whole birds, and more. Bone-in, boneless. Skin-on, skinless. A quick scan of your supermarket's refrigerated poultry section, not to mention the freezer section, reveals just how many poultry choices you have. All parts provide complete protein with a limited amount of saturated fat.

If you're looking for a lean protein source, pick up a package of skinless breast meat. You'll save 12 milligrams sodium choosing boneless, skinless breast meat over the same serving size of dark meat from a broiler-fryer (63 milligrams versus 75 milligrams). The difference is greater in a stewing chicken, with the dark meat containing nearly twice as much sodium as the light meat.

> **PINCH OF SAGE**
>
> A serving size of poultry is 3 ounces, which is about the size of a deck of cards. Chicken breast halves packaged in the supermarket are often heavier, though. After cooking, you might want to divide them into appropriate portions. If you do eat a larger chicken breast half, be sure to calculate the additional sodium, as well as calories, protein, fat, and so on.

No matter what your poultry-part preference, pass on the skin and deep-frying. You don't need either to prepare a well-seasoned poultry dish. Because you're flavoring without shaking on salt or other high-sodium seasonings and sauces, the skinless pieces allow those tastes to come through even better.

Skin-on birds, such as Cornish game hens and young chickens, and parts, such as thighs and drumsticks, may be your only options in your store's poultry section. If that's the case, remove the skin before cooking. Or you can discard it before serving. Cooking poultry with the skin on doesn't add any fat to the meat, but it does hold in the juices for better flavor. If a recipe calls for removing the skin prior to cooking, do so before boning the poultry to make the job easier.

Better Safe Than Sorry

Thinking about all the delicious, low-sodium poultry dishes you can create may make you want to toss a few choice packages into your shopping cart. Stop! Poultry may be nearly perfect, but it does associate with some nasty bacteria so you must take care when handling it.

In the store, keep any raw juices from contaminating your hands or other groceries. Use the plastic disposable bags available to enclose your poultry picks. (If these bags aren't located in the meat department, take a few from the produce section.) Slip your hand into the bag wrong side out, choose your poultry, and turn the bag right side out over the package. Hit the checkout next, and make a beeline for your house (storing your poultry in a cooler in your trunk if you have a lengthy drive), storing your purchases in the refrigerator or freezer ASAP.

Thawing poultry in the refrigerator or microwave is easy. Allow 3 or 4 hours per pound for defrosting a whole bird in the refrigerator; parts require less time. Follow the manufacturer's directions for your microwave, and cook the poultry immediately. You also may thaw waterproof packages by submerging them in cold water, but be sure to change the water every 30 minutes to keep it cold.

While preparing poultry, wash your hands every time before you touch something else. Using separate utensils, cutting boards, dishes, and pans for raw poultry also keeps cross-contamination at bay.

Cook your birds until the juices run clear, and check the internal temperature with a thermometer. See the following table for suggested temperatures.

Temperature Guidelines

Poultry Type	Recommended Cooked Temperature
All whole chickens or turkeys	180°F
Thighs, wings, or legs	180°F
Breasts or roasts	170°F
Ground chicken or turkey	165°F

Skillet-Sizzled Herb-Buttered Turkey

This quick-fix entrée serves up turkey breast coated with a paprika-tinged buttery sauce with fresh basil, parsley, and tarragon flavors.

Yield:	Prep time:	Cook time:	Serving size:
4 servings	2 minutes	10 minutes	3 ounces cooked turkey breast

Each serving has:		
211 calories	41.6 mg sodium	

1 recipe Herb-Flecked Butter (recipe in Chapter 14)	$\frac{1}{8}$ tsp. garlic powder
$\frac{1}{4}$ tsp. paprika	1 lb. turkey breast fillets

1. Place Herb-Flecked Butter, paprika, and garlic powder in a small microwave-safe bowl, and cook on high for 1 minute or just until melted. Stir.

2. Heat a large nonstick skillet over medium heat. When hot, add turkey fillets, and sear for 1 minute. Turn and sear on the other side for 1 minute.

3. Using a pastry brush, brush half of butter mixture over turkey fillets. Turn and brush remaining butter mixture over the other side. Cover and cook for 8 to 10 minutes or until a food thermometer reads 170°F.

4. Cut into equal portions as necessary before serving.

PINCH OF SAGE

To check the internal temperature of your meats accurately, remember to position the tip of the meat thermometer in the middle of a thick, meaty portion without touching a bone or piercing through to touch the pan.

Plum Delicious Chicken

Tender baked chicken breasts are topped with an Asian-inspired plum sauce.

Yield:	Prep time:	Cook time:	Serving size:
4 servings	15 minutes	25 minutes	1 chicken breast half with about ⅓ cup sauce

Each serving has:	
157 calories	43.8 mg sodium

4 (3-oz.) boneless, skinless chicken breast halves, trimmed, rinsed, and patted dry with paper towels

½ cup heavy syrup from ready-to-serve prunes

½ tsp. ground ginger

3 medium cloves garlic, minced

1 TB. fresh lemon juice

¾ cup ready-to-serve prunes (about 12 to 14), pitted and quartered

1. Preheat the oven to 350°F. Lightly spray a 2-quart glass baking dish with nonstick cooking spray.

2. Arrange chicken in the prepared baking dish.

3. In a small bowl, combine heavy syrup from prunes, ginger, garlic, and lemon juice. Add prunes, and pour sauce over chicken.

4. Cover and bake for 25 minutes or until cooked through, no longer pink, and juices run clear.

PINCH OF SAGE

The flavor of fresh lemon juice is superior, but if you can't get fresh lemons, use bottled lemon juice. Because you're depending on flavorings other than salt, you might consider keeping fresh lemons on hand.

Oven-Fried Chicken

Well-seasoned, whole-wheat flour breads oven-baked chicken breasts for the taste of fried chicken.

Yield:	Prep time:	Cook time:	Serving size:
4 chicken breast halves	15 minutes	20 minutes	1 chicken breast half
Each serving has:			
129 calories	45.4 mg sodium		

1/4 cup whole-wheat flour

1 tsp. dried thyme

3/4 tsp. Salt-Shaker Substitute (recipe in Chapter 14)

1/2 tsp. freshly ground black pepper

1/2 tsp. dried oregano

1/4 tsp. garlic powder

1/8 tsp. dried crushed rosemary

1/8 tsp. paprika

2 TB. fat-free milk

4 (3-oz.) boneless skinless chicken breast halves, trimmed, rinsed, and patted dry with paper towels

Nonstick cooking spray

1. Adjust the oven rack to the upper-middle position, and preheat the oven to 400°F. Line a baking sheet with aluminum foil, place a wire rack on the baking sheet, and spray it with nonstick cooking spray.

2. In a shallow dish, combine whole-wheat flour, thyme, Salt-Shaker Substitute, pepper, oregano, garlic powder, rosemary, and paprika, and stir to blend well.

3. Pour milk into another shallow dish.

4. Dip each chicken breast half into milk, allowing excess to drip off, and dredge in seasoned flour, coating completely and gently shaking off excess. Place chicken upside down on the rack. Spray undersides of chicken with nonstick cooking spray, turn over, and spray tops, coating completely.

5. Bake for 20 to 25 minutes or until cooked through, no longer pink, and juices run clear.

Salternative: Use your favorite savory salt-free seasoning blend instead of the Salt-Shaker Substitute, if you prefer.

> **PINCH OF SAGE**
>
> When Herbert Hoover used the phrase "a chicken in every pot" during his 1928 presidential campaign, he promised prosperity and well-being. Beyond being a healthful choice, chicken, as well as turkey, is an economical option.

Tropical Chicken for Two

Thin-pounded chicken breasts are served in a sweet pineapple sauce seasoned with cinnamon, oregano, and parsley.

Yield:	Prep time:	Cook time:	Serving size:
2 servings	10 minutes	15 minutes	1 chicken breast half with $\frac{1}{2}$ of sauce

Each serving has:			
208 calories	45.6 mg sodium		

2 (3-oz.) boneless skinless chicken breast halves, trimmed, rinsed, and patted dry with paper towels	1 TB. extra-light olive oil
	$\frac{3}{4}$ cup pineapple juice
	1 TB. fresh lime juice
$\frac{1}{4}$ tsp. dried oregano	1 tsp. cornstarch
$\frac{1}{8}$ tsp. ground cinnamon	1 tsp. dried parsley flakes

1. Place chicken between 2 sheets of waxed paper. Using the flat side of a meat mallet or a rolling pin, pound chicken to a $\frac{1}{2}$-inch thickness. Sprinkle $\frac{1}{2}$ of oregano and $\frac{1}{2}$ of cinnamon over chicken.

2. In a large skillet over medium heat, heat extra-light olive oil. Add chicken, seasoned side down, and sprinkle remaining oregano and cinnamon over chicken. Cook for 5 minutes. Turn and cook for 5 more minutes or until cooked through, no longer pink, and juices run clear. Remove chicken to a serving platter.

3. In a small bowl, stir together pineapple juice, lime juice, and cornstarch. Pour into the skillet, and bring to a boil over medium to medium-high heat. Stir almost constantly until thickened.

4. Stir in parsley flakes, and spoon sauce over chicken to serve.

PINCH OF SAGE

Fresh herbs do nicely as salt substitutions. If a recipe calls for 1 teaspoon dried herb, use 1 tablespoon fresh. Drying decreases the volume of the herb, so you need more fresh herb to get the same flavor. In this recipe, substitute ¾ teaspoon chopped fresh oregano and 1 tablespoon chopped fresh parsley.

Stovetop Cranberry Chicken

Lightly coated chicken breasts are topped with tangy cranberry sauce and served over brown rice.

Yield:	Prep time:	Cook time:	Serving size:
4 servings	10 minutes	35 minutes	½ cup rice with 1 chicken breast half and ¼ sauce

Each serving has:	
403 calories	57.2 mg sodium

⅓ cup whole-wheat flour

¼ tsp. freshly ground black pepper

1½ TB. extra-light olive oil

4 (3-oz.) boneless, skinless chicken breast halves, trimmed, rinsed, and patted dry with paper towels

1 cup water

1 cup fresh or frozen cranberries

½ cup firmly packed light brown sugar

Dash nutmeg

1 TB. red wine vinegar

2 cups cooked long-grain brown rice

1. In a shallow dish, stir together whole-wheat flour and pepper.

2. In a large deep skillet over medium heat, heat extra-light olive oil.

3. *Dredge* chicken in seasoned flour, coating it completely, and add to the skillet. Brown chicken for 3 or 4 minutes on both sides, remove from the skillet, and keep warm.

4. Remove the skillet from heat. Pour in water and cranberries, and return to heat. Stir in light brown sugar, nutmeg, and red wine vinegar. Cook, stirring often, for 5 minutes or until cranberries burst. Return chicken to the skillet.

5. Reduce heat, cover, and simmer for 20 minutes or until chicken is cooked through, no longer pink, and juices run clear. Serve each chicken breast half on a bed of rice, spooning sauce over all.

Salternative: If you're short on time or haven't cooked the rice ahead of time, substitute instant brown rice. Remember that instant rices contain some sodium, though, ranging from 5 to 20 milligrams.

DEFINITION

Dredge is the motion of moving a moist or moistened food through a dry substance, such as seasoned flour, to coat the food.

Grilled Asian-Spiced Chicken Thighs

Rich-flavored chicken thighs are dredged in a spicy-sweet coating that serves as a marinade and a grilling sauce.

Yield:	Prep time:	Chill time:	Cook time:	Serving size:
12 chicken thighs	15 minutes	30 minutes	10 minutes	2 chicken thighs

Each serving has:				
237 calories	91 mg sodium			

2 TB. Asian-Inspired Spice Blend (recipe in Chapter 14)

2 TB. honey

3 lb. chicken thighs, skin and bones removed, rinsed, and patted dry with paper towels

1. In a shallow bowl, combine Asian-Inspired Spice Blend and honey, mixing thoroughly.

2. Lightly coat chicken by dredging both sides in honey mixture. Arrange chicken on a baking sheet or tray, and marinate in the refrigerator for at least 30 minutes.

3. Generously coat the grill rack with nonstick spray. Preheat grill to high.

4. Arrange chicken on grill rack, cover, and grill for 10 minutes or until cooked through, no longer pink, and juices run clear, turning and rotating after 5 minutes.

PINCH OF SAGE

Never marinate meat on the kitchen counter. Dangerous bacteria can multiply quickly at room temperature. Always marinate meat in the refrigerator.

Saucy Orange Chicken over Angel Hair

Sweet bell peppers top chicken breasts baked in an Asian-flavored orange sauce.

Yield:	Prep time:	Cook time:	Serving size:
4 servings	20 minutes	35 minutes	$\frac{1}{2}$ cup pasta with 1 chicken breast half and $\frac{1}{4}$ sauce

Each serving has:	
271 calories	99.6 mg sodium

4 (3-oz.) boneless skinless chicken breast halves, trimmed, rinsed, and patted dry with paper towels

1 cup unsweetened orange juice

1 tsp. *lite soy sauce*

2 TB. firmly packed light brown sugar

$\frac{1}{2}$ tsp. ground dry mustard

$\frac{1}{4}$ tsp. ground ginger

1 tsp. dried basil

1 TB. grated orange zest

$\frac{1}{2}$ cup sliced green onions (about 4)

$\frac{1}{2}$ large green bell pepper, ribs and seeds removed, and cut into thin strips

$\frac{1}{2}$ large red bell pepper, ribs and seeds removed, and cut into thin strips

1 TB. cornstarch

2 TB. fresh lemon juice

2 cups cooked angel hair pasta

1. Preheat the oven to 350°F. Lightly spray the bottom of a 13×9×2-inch glassware baking dish with nonstick cooking spray.

2. Arrange chicken breast halves in the prepared dish.

3. In a small bowl, combine orange juice and lite soy sauce. Whisk in light brown sugar, dry mustard, ginger, basil, and orange zest until well combined. Pour over chicken.

4. Scatter green onions, green bell pepper, and red bell pepper over chicken. Cover the dish tightly with aluminum foil, and bake for 30 minutes or until chicken is cooked through, no longer pink, and juices run clear.

5. In a small bowl, whisk together cornstarch and lemon juice. Stir into sauce around chicken. Bake for 5 more minutes or until sauce thickens slightly.

6. To serve, mound cooked pasta on a serving platter and arrange chicken on top. Scatter some onions and peppers over chicken, and spoon some sauce over all. Serve remaining sauce on the side.

Salternative: If you can afford the added sodium, this dish is also nice served over a bed of rice noodles. The sodium content varies among brands, so check the nutrition labels.

> **DEFINITION**
>
> **Lite soy sauce** is lower in sodium than regular soy sauce. If you have regular soy sauce, substitute a mixture of ½ regular soy sauce and ½ water for the lite soy sauce. Depending on the brand, this might cut down on the sodium.

Tasty Turkey-Stuffed Peppers

Ground turkey breast, brown rice, and seasoned tomato sauce fill tender green bell peppers.

Yield:	Prep time:	Cook time:	Serving size:
4 stuffed bell pepper halves	15 minutes	55 minutes	1 stuffed bell pepper half
Each serving has:			
249 calories	110 mg sodium		

2 large green bell peppers, ribs and seeds removed, and halved lengthwise

1 lb. ground turkey breast or ground turkey

½ cup uncooked instant brown rice

1 (8-oz.) can no-salt-added tomato sauce

½ cup finely grated carrots

¼ cup diced onions

2 medium cloves garlic, minced

3 TB. chopped fresh parsley

1 tsp. dried oregano

½ tsp. Salt-Shaker Substitute (recipe in Chapter 14) or other salt-free salt substitute seasoning blend

½ tsp. freshly ground black pepper

1. Preheat the oven to 350°F. Lightly spray the bottom of a 2-quart glassware baking dish with nonstick cooking spray.

2. Place green bell pepper halves in the prepared baking dish.

3. In a medium bowl, combine ground turkey breast, instant brown rice, tomato sauce, carrots, onions, garlic, parsley, oregano, Salt-Shaker Substitute, and pepper. Mix well.

4. Spoon mixture into green bell pepper halves. Cover with nonstick aluminum foil, and bake for 55 to 60 minutes or until cooked through and turkey is no longer pink.

PINCH OF SAGE

If you have only regular aluminum foil, lightly spray the sheet with nonstick cooking spray and place it sprayed side down over the baking dish.

Thai Chicken Basil Balls over Jasmine Rice

Sweet basil flavors these chicken meatballs served with a sweet-tart lime sauce, all with an undertone of chili-pepper heat.

Yield:	Prep time:	Cook time:	Serving size:
4 servings	15 minutes	26 minutes	6 meatballs with 2 tablespoons sauce and ½ cup rice

Each serving has:			
362.2 calories	112.8 mg sodium		

1 TB. sesame seed oil	1 tsp. grated lime zest
4 medium serrano chili peppers or other hot peppers to taste, ribs and seeds removed, and minced	⅓ cup fresh lime juice
	2 TB. Sodium-Wise Soy Sauce Stand-In (recipe in Chapter 12)
¼ cup minced red onions	½ tsp. *hot chili oil* or to taste
5 medium cloves garlic, minced	1 tsp. firmly packed light brown sugar
1 TB. peeled and minced gingerroot	1 TB. chopped fresh basil
½ cup coarsely chopped fresh basil	2 cups cooked jasmine rice
1 lb. ground chicken breast	

1. Preheat the oven to 400°F.

2. Heat a small nonstick skillet over medium-low heat. When hot, add sesame seed oil. Stir in serrano chili peppers and red onions, and cook, stirring occasionally, for 5 minutes or until onions are translucent.

3. Stir in garlic and gingerroot, and cook, stirring frequently, for 2 minutes. Stir in ½ cup coarsely chopped basil and cook, stirring, for 1 minute or until basil is wilted.

4. In a large bowl, combine ground chicken breast and chili pepper mixture. Shape into 24 (1½-inch) balls, and arrange on a large nonstick baking sheet. Bake for 18 to 20 minutes or until a food thermometer reads 165°F.

5. Meanwhile, in a small bowl, combine lime zest, lime juice, Sodium-Wise Soy Sauce Stand-In, hot chili oil, light brown sugar, and remaining 1 tablespoon basil. Whisk to blend.

6. To serve, line each serving plate with ½ cup jasmine rice. Top with 6 meatballs, and drizzle 2 tablespoons lime juice mixture over all.

Salternative: Substitute Thai chili peppers and Thai basil in equal amounts, if you have access to these ingredients.

> **DEFINITION**
>
> **Hot chili oil** is a fiery infusion made with a blend of vegetable oils and dried red chili peppers. Look for it in your supermarket's Asian foods section. Remember to shake well before using because the chili peppers tend to settle to the bottom.

Turkey Medallions with Sun-Dried Tomatoes

Skillet-sizzled turkey breast is sauced with bright-tasting green onions and rich sun-dried tomatoes.

Yield:	Prep time:	Cook time:	Serving size:
6 servings	20 minutes	10 minutes	4 ounces turkey with ¼ cup sauce

Each serving has:		
174 calories	156.8 mg sodium	

½ cup dry-packed sun-dried tomatoes	¼ tsp. ground white pepper
1½ lb. turkey breast tenderloins, rinsed and patted dry with paper towels	2 TB. extra-light olive oil
	½ cup chopped green onions

1. Pack sun-dried tomatoes in a 1-cup measuring cup. Pour enough hot water over tomatoes to fill the measuring cup, and let tomatoes stand for at least 10 minutes or until softened. Slice tomatoes, reserving liquid.

2. Slice turkey into ¾-inch-thick medallions, and season with white pepper.

3. In a large skillet over medium to medium-high heat, heat extra-light olive oil. Add turkey medallions, and sauté for 3 minutes on each side or until cooked through, no longer pink, and juices run clear. Using a slotted spatula, remove medallions to a paper towel–lined plate and blot dry. Reduce heat to medium-low.

4. Add green onions to the same skillet, and sauté for 1 minute. Add tomatoes and reserved liquid, and cook for 2 or 3 minutes or until heated through.

5. To serve, transfer medallions to a serving platter, and spoon sauce over top.

PINCH OF SAGE

Cooking the turkey medallions over medium-high heat seals in the juices for a flavorful meal. However, sautéing at this temperature creates splattering. Put the skillet on a back burner, use a spatter guard if you have one, and wear an oven mitt to prevent burns while you turn the turkey.

Creamy Dilled Turkey Cutlets with Vegetables

Dill-flavored turkey breast joins broccoli, corn, and spinach in a tangy yogurt sauce.

Yield:	Prep time:	Cook time:	Serving size:
4 servings	5 minutes	15 minutes	3 ounces cooked turkey with $\frac{1}{2}$ cup sauce

Each serving has:	
186 calories	160.4 mg sodium

$\frac{1}{2}$ TB. extra-light olive oil

1 lb. turkey cutlets, rinsed and patted dry with paper towels

1 tsp. dried dill weed

$\frac{1}{2}$ tsp. Salt-Shaker Substitute (recipe in Chapter 14) or other savory salt-free salt substitute seasoning blend

$\frac{1}{4}$ tsp. freshly ground black pepper

1 cup frozen broccoli florets

$\frac{1}{2}$ cup frozen corn kernels

$\frac{1}{2}$ cup frozen cut spinach

1 cup fat-free plain yogurt

1. In a large skillet over medium heat, heat extra-light olive oil. Add turkey, and sauté for 3 minutes. Turn and sauté on other side for 2 more minutes while sprinkling on dill weed, Salt-Shaker Substitute, and pepper.

2. Add broccoli, corn, and spinach. Cover and cook for 6 minutes or until vegetables are tender and turkey is cooked through, no longer pink, and juices run clear.

3. Remove the skillet from heat. Stir in yogurt, blending well.

4. Return to low heat, cover, and cook for 2 minutes or until heated through. (Do not boil.)

Salternative: You can substitute 2 cups of your favorite plain frozen veggies in this recipe instead of the broccoli, corn, and spinach called for.

SALT PITFALL

Frozen peas are processed with salt and are, therefore, significantly higher in sodium than other frozen vegetables.

Savory Chicken with Green Beans and Mushrooms

Sage- and thyme-coated chicken breasts are baked with sautéed mushrooms and green beans and seasoned with cloves.

Yield:	Prep time:	Cook time:	Serving size:
4 servings	10 minutes	50 minutes	1 chicken breast half with 1 cup vegetables

Each serving has:	
271 calories	174 mg sodium

1/3 cup whole-wheat flour
1/2 tsp. dried rubbed sage
1/2 tsp. dried thyme
3 TB. extra-light olive oil
4 (3-oz.) boneless, skinless chicken breast halves, trimmed, rinsed, and patted dry with paper towels

3/4 tsp. ground cloves
8 oz. sliced button mushrooms
1 (16-oz.) pkg. frozen cut green beans, thawed and drained

1. Preheat the oven to 400°F. Lightly spray the bottom of a 9×9×2-inch glass baking dish with nonstick cooking spray.

2. In a shallow bowl, stir together whole-wheat flour, sage, and thyme.

3. In a large ovenproof skillet over medium heat, heat 2 tablespoons extra-light olive oil.

4. Dredge chicken in seasoned flour to coat completely, and add to the skillet. Brown chicken on both sides, transfer to the prepared baking dish, and lightly sprinkle cloves over top.

5. In a medium skillet over medium-low heat, heat remaining 1 tablespoon olive oil. Add mushrooms, and sauté for 5 minutes or until colored.

6. In the large skillet, sauté green beans, dusting with any remaining seasoned flour, and cook for 3 minutes. Stir in mushrooms, and spoon green beans and mushrooms over chicken.

7. Cover and bake for 30 to 40 minutes or until chicken is cooked through, no longer pink, and juices run clear, and sauce is formed.

PINCH OF SAGE

Fresh or thawed chicken breast halves can sometimes be difficult to trim with a knife. Using your fingers to grasp and pull off the fat deposits may be easier. Just be certain to wash your hands thoroughly before and especially after.

Indian-Inspired Curried Chicken with Golden Raisins

A golden curry sauce smothers bite-size chicken thigh pieces and sweet, plumped golden raisins while topping nutty brown rice.

Yield:	Prep time:	Cook time:	Serving size:
7 servings	3 minutes	22 minutes	½ cup curry with ½ cup rice

Each serving has:	
344 calories	232.1 mg sodium

¼ cup extra-virgin olive oil

4 tsp. salt-free curry powder

¼ cup all-purpose flour

3 cups reduced-sodium, fat-free chicken broth

¾ cup golden raisins

2 cups (½-in.-cubed) cooked chicken thighs

1 TB. Salt-Shaker Substitute (recipe in Chapter 14) or other salt-free salt substitute seasoning blend

¼ tsp. freshly ground black pepper

3½ cups cooked brown rice

1. Heat a large skillet over medium-low heat. When hot, add extra-virgin olive oil, and heat for 1 minute. Stir in curry powder and flour until blended, and cook for 3 minutes or until bubbly and thickened.

2. Slowly stir in chicken broth until blended. Add raisins. Increase heat to medium, and bring to a simmer. Simmer for 10 minutes, stirring occasionally, or until sauce is thickened and raisins are tender.

3. Stir in chicken, Salt-Shaker Substitute, and pepper. Cook for 2 minutes or until heated through.

4. Spoon curry mixture over brown rice to serve.

PINCH OF SAGE

If you're unsure of the salt content of commercial-brand curry powders, you can mix your own blend. Combine 2 tablespoons ground cumin, 1½ tablespoons ground coriander, 1 tablespoon ground turmeric, 1 teaspoon ground ginger, ¼ teaspoon cayenne, and ¼ teaspoon paprika. Other additions might include cardamom, fennel seeds, mustard seeds, fenugreek, black pepper, cloves, and/or cinnamon—all well ground.

Big Beef and Prime Pork

In This Chapter

- Keeping your kitchen safe
- Making meats a healthful choice
- Low-sodium beef favorites
- Working with the "other white meat"

When they sit down to dinner, many families expect to find meat on their plates. If this is the case at your house, you might have found yourself staring at a package of ground beef, wondering how to prepare it now that salt is out. The good news is that the bold flavor of beef and pork can deliciously take on thick, rich, deep flavors that satisfy—without sodium.

With just a few substitutions and cooking hints, you can put the meat back on the dinner table, taking your pick from an array of cuts to fit a variety of budgets and any number of occasions. Use the recipes in this chapter to get you started, and take the secrets back to your family-favorite recipes.

Safe at Home

You've brought home your meat selections, wrapped in plastic bags to avoid cross-contamination. You've immediately stored them on the lowest shelf of your refrigerator, below any foods to be served raw so in case the meat drips, the liquid won't affect any raw foods in your refrigerator.

When the time comes to cook your beef or pork (within 3 or 4 days), you use separate cutting boards, utensils, and dishes for the raw meat, and you wash your hands before and after handling the meat. You've done everything to make the meal safe, right?

So far, yes, you have. But you're not done. When you think you're finished cooking, how do you know if the meat is done? It's brown on the inside so you can serve it, right? Maybe.

You can't tell if meats, especially ground meats, are thoroughly cooked just by sight. Although beef and pork cuts may be served medium rare or medium, ground meats must be thoroughly cooked. During the grinding process, surface bacteria such as E. coli are introduced into the meat. E. coli is not killed at refrigerator or freezer temperatures, but only through careful cooking.

The only certain test to determine if meats are safe to eat is the internal temperature. Use a meat thermometer every time. Insert the thermometer into the thickest part of the meat, being sure the thermometer doesn't rest on a bone or pass through the meat and touch the pan. Remember to wash the meat thermometer like any other utensil in hot, soapy water after every use. The following table gives recommended temperatures for beef and pork.

Temperature Guidelines

Meat	Recommended Cooked Temperature
Ground beef, pork, and veal	160°F
Beef	
Medium rare	145°F
Medium	160°F
Well done	170°F
Pork	
Medium	160°F
Well done	170°F

Helpful Hints

At times, beef and pork have been maligned for their fatty nature, but don't let that stop you. Just choose lean cuts of meat. Plus, trimming any visible fat keeps your intake at reasonable levels.

The recipes in this chapter call for 85-percent-lean ground beef because it's commonly available and inexpensive. Certainly, you can substitute 92-percent-lean or another leaner ground beef if you like. Although you won't want to add any fat back in with cooking oils, you may need to spray the pan with nonstick cooking spray to facilitate cooking.

Many beef and pork recipes call for breadcrumbs or cracker crumbs as coatings and fillers. Salt-free breadcrumbs and coating mixes are available, but sometimes they're difficult to find. Readily available sodium-free substitutions enable you to enjoy your favorite recipes again. Quick oats work well as a filler. And unsalted matzo meal makes a good coating; look for it in the ethnic aisle of your supermarket.

Indian Nectar Pork Chops

Curried apricot nectar infuses flavor into everyday pork chops.

Yield:	Prep time:	Cook time:	Serving size:
4 pork chops	5 minutes	25 minutes	1 pork chop

Each serving has:		
269 calories	52 mg sodium	

1 TB. extra-light olive oil	¼ tsp. garlic powder
4 (½-in.-thick) pork loin chops	¼ tsp. Salt-Shaker Substitute (recipe in Chapter 14) or other salt-free salt substitute seasoning blend
¾ cup apricot nectar	
1 tsp. salt-free curry powder	

1. In a large, nonstick skillet over medium-high heat, heat extra-light olive oil. Add pork chops, and brown for 2 or 3 minutes on both sides.

2. In a measuring cup, whisk together apricot nectar, curry powder, garlic powder, and Salt-Shaker Substitute.

3. Pour apricot nectar mixture over pork chops, and bring to a simmer. Reduce heat as needed to maintain a simmer, and simmer, uncovered, for 10 minutes. Turn pork chops, and simmer for 10 more minutes or until done (170°F on a food thermometer).

PINCH OF SAGE

Serve these quick and easy pork chops with whole-wheat couscous or brown rice for an enjoyable meal.

Onion-Smothered Pork Chops

Savory, highly seasoned onions accompany every bite of these simply stovetop-cooked pork chops.

Yield:	Prep time:	Cook time:	Serving size:
4 pork chops	5 minutes	30 minutes	1 pork chop with 2 tablespoons onions

Each serving has:	
259.4 calories	52.9 mg sodium

1 TB. extra-light olive oil	2 tsp. freshly ground black pepper
4 (½-in.-thick) pork loin chops	1 medium yellow onion, halved and sliced
3 tsp. Salt-Shaker Substitute (recipe in Chapter 14) or other salt-free salt substitute seasoning blend	1 cup water

1. In a large nonstick skillet over medium heat, heat extra-light olive oil.

2. Rub pork chops with 2 teaspoons Salt-Shaker Substitute and 1 teaspoon pepper. Add pork chops to the skillet, and brown on both sides.

3. Add onion and water, reduce heat as needed to maintain a simmer, cover, and simmer for 20 minutes.

4. Turn pork chops, and season with remaining 1 teaspoon Salt-Shaker Substitute and remaining 1 teaspoon pepper. Uncover and cook for 5 to 10 more minutes or until liquid is evaporated and onions are golden.

Salternative: Reduce the amount of black pepper if you prefer a less-spicy flavor.

PINCH OF SAGE

For optimal shelf life, purchase olive oil in a tin or dark bottle and store it in a cool, dark place tightly sealed. Light and heat shortens its lifespan.

Rosemary-Crusted Pork Tenderloin

Tender, slow-cooked pork tenderloin is crusted with a savory seasoning mix.

Yield:	Prep time:	Cook time:	Serving size:
6 to 8 servings	10 minutes	2 hours	3 ounces cooked pork

Each serving has:		
153.8 calories	57.3 mg sodium	

1 cup water	2 tsp. extra-light olive oil
1 tsp. freshly ground black pepper	3 medium cloves garlic, crushed
1 (1½- to 2-lb.) pkg. pork tenderloins	2 tsp. dried crushed rosemary

1. Preheat the oven to 350°F. Spray the rack of a roasting pan with nonstick cooking spray.

2. Pour water into the bottom of the prepared roasting pan.

3. Spread pepper on a sheet of waxed paper.

4. Brush surface of pork tenderloins with extra-light olive oil. Rub on garlic, sprinkle on rosemary, and roll in pepper, keeping tenderloins' rolled shape.

5. Place pork tenderloins on the rack in the prepared roasting pan, cover, and roast for 2 hours or until it reaches an internal temperature of 160°F.

PINCH OF SAGE

The garlic is very pungent while the meat roasts, but the flavor is mild in the finished tenderloin.

Fiery Steak with Southwestern Relish

Spicy seasoned rib-eye is broiled and served with fresh tomato, corn, and avocado relish.

Yield:	Prep time:	Cook time:	Serving size:
4 servings	5 minutes	10 minutes	3 ounces cooked steak with $\frac{1}{3}$ cup relish

Each serving has:			
312.3 calories	59.3 mg sodium		

1 lb. thin-cut boneless rib-eye beef steaks

1 tsp. salt-free *garlic-pepper blend*

1 tsp. Firehouse Chili Powder (recipe in Chapter 14) or other salt-free chili powder blend

1$\frac{1}{3}$ cups Southwestern Relish (recipe in Chapter 13)

1. Preheat the broiler to high. Spray the rack of a broiler pan with nonstick cooking spray.

2. Place steaks on the broiler pan. Season both sides with garlic-pepper blend and Firehouse Chili Powder. Broil for 5 minutes. Turn and broil other side for 5 minutes or until done as desired (160°F for medium).

3. Serve with Southwestern Relish.

DEFINITION

Garlic-pepper blend is a mixture of garlic, black pepper, bell peppers, and onions. Different blends contain various seasonings—and sometimes salt—so read labels carefully.

After-Work Chili Mac

Italian-seasoned tomato sauce coats whole-wheat rotini, ground beef, corn, bell peppers, and onions.

Yield:	Prep time:	Cook time:	Serving size:
6 cups	5 minutes	12 minutes	1½ cups

Each serving has:			
469.6 calories	71.4 mg sodium		

¾ lb. 85-percent-lean ground beef

1 small yellow onion, diced

½ medium green bell pepper, ribs and seeds removed, and diced

1 tsp. Salt-Shaker Substitute (recipe in Chapter 14) or other savory salt-free salt substitute seasoning blend

½ tsp. Italian seasoning

2½ cups whole-wheat rotini pasta

1 (8-oz.) can no-salt-added tomato sauce

1 cup water

1 cup frozen whole-kernel corn

1. In a deep, medium nonstick skillet over medium heat, cook ground beef, onion, green bell pepper, Salt-Shaker Substitute, and Italian seasoning. Cook and stir, breaking up meat, for 5 to 8 minutes or until beef is browned. Drain grease from the skillet.

2. Meanwhile, cook pasta according to the package directions (omit salt). Drain.

3. Add tomato sauce, water, and corn to the skillet. Bring to a boil, and reduce heat as needed to maintain a simmer. Cover and simmer for 5 minutes or until corn is cooked.

4. Stir in pasta, and heat through.

Salternative: If you can afford the additional sodium, sprinkle on a little shredded low-sodium cheddar cheese.

PINCH OF SAGE

You can measure the 1 cup water by filling the empty tomato sauce can because 8 ounces equals 1 cup. This method saves the time of scraping the can clean.

Stir-Fried Sweet-and-Sour Pork

Bite-size pork, onions, green bell peppers, and pineapple are immersed in a tasty sweet-and-sour sauce.

Yield:	Prep time:	Cook time:	Serving size:
5 cups	3 minutes	11 minutes	1¼ cups
Each serving has:			
324.2 calories	81.9 mg sodium		

1 (20-oz.) can pineapple chunks packed in juice, drained (¾ cup juice reserved)	1 lb. trimmed pork loin, chops, tenderloin, or stew meat, cut into 1-in. cubes
3 TB. Sodium-Wise Soy Sauce Stand-In (recipe in Chapter 12)	1 cup coarsely chopped onions
1 TB. cider vinegar	1 cup coarsely chopped green bell peppers
1 TB. firmly packed light brown sugar	2 medium cloves garlic, minced
1 TB. cornstarch	1 TB. peeled and minced gingerroot

1. In a measuring cup or a small bowl, combine reserved pineapple juice, Sodium-Wise Soy Sauce Stand-In, cider vinegar, and light brown sugar. Whisk to blend. Add cornstarch, and whisk to blend. Set aside.

2. Heat a nonstick wok or a large skillet over medium-high heat. When hot, add pork cubes, and stir-fry for 3 minutes or until browned on all sides.

3. Add onions, green bell peppers, pineapple chunks, garlic, and gingerroot, and stir-fry for 6 to 8 minutes or until vegetables are crisp-tender.

4. Whisk pineapple juice mixture, and pour into the wok. Continue stir-frying for 2 minutes or until heated through and pork temperature reads 170°F on a food thermometer.

5. Serve over hot cooked rice or wheat or rice noodles, as desired.

PINCH OF SAGE

If your pork is particularly lean, you may want to add a small amount of canola or peanut oil to the wok before adding pork to facilitate stir-frying. If using, however, keep the oil addition to a minimum because you just want the foods to stir easily and not end up with an oily sauce.

Grilled T-Bones with Charred Peppers

Lime-marinated T-bone steaks are grilled and served alongside colorful roasted sweet peppers.

Yield:	Prep time:	Chill time:	Cook time:	Serving size:
4 servings	20 minutes	8 hours	25 minutes	3 ounces cooked steak with ¾ cup bell peppers

Each serving has:	
407.2 calories	92.3 mg sodium

Grated zest of 1 medium lime	¼ tsp. freshly ground black pepper
Juice of 1 medium lime	2 lb. tailless T-bone steaks
1 medium clove garlic, crushed	1 medium green bell pepper
2 tsp. dried oregano	1 medium red bell pepper
1½ TB. extra-virgin olive oil	1 medium yellow bell pepper

1. In a large zipper-lock bag, combine lime zest, lime juice, garlic, oregano, extra-virgin olive oil, and pepper. Add steaks, seal the bag, and turn to coat well. Marinate in the refrigerator for 8 hours or overnight.

2. Preheat the grill to low. Spray the rack with nonstick grilling spray.

3. Place green bell pepper, red bell pepper, and yellow bell pepper on the grill rack, close lid, and cook for 10 minutes or until blackened and charred on all sides, turning gently with tongs. Remove to a zipper-lock bag. Seal and steam for 10 minutes.

4. Remove steaks from marinade, and discard marinade. Add steaks to the grill rack, close lid, and cook for 10 minutes. Turn and cook, with lid closed, for 5 minutes on other side or until done as desired (160°F for medium). Remove to a serving platter. Let stand for a few minutes before serving.

5. Meanwhile, peel skins from bell peppers, and discard seeds and cap. Cut peppers into strips, and serve with steaks.

PINCH OF SAGE

The bell peppers may be too hot to handle when you first remove them from the bag. Wait a minute until you can comfortably handle them. It'll be easier to peel the skins then as well.

Maple-Barbecue Country-Style Pork Ribs

Slow-baked spareribs are basted with a maple-flavored tomato-based barbecue sauce.

Yield:	Prep time:	Cook time:	Serving size:
6 servings	20 minutes	1 hour, 40 minutes	3 ounces cooked meat

Each serving has:	
520.9 calories	89 mg sodium

1½ lb. boneless country-style pork spareribs

1 cup unsweetened applesauce

1 cup pure maple syrup

½ cup no-salt-added ketchup

6 TB. fresh lemon juice

¼ tsp. ground cinnamon

¼ tsp. paprika

¼ tsp. garlic powder

¼ tsp. Salt-Shaker Substitute (recipe in Chapter 14) or other salt-free salt substitute seasoning blend

¼ tsp. freshly ground black pepper

1. Preheat the oven to 325°F. Spray an 8×8-inch baking pan with nonstick cooking spray.

2. Place spareribs in a large pan. Cover with water, and bring to a boil over high heat. Reduce heat to low, and simmer for 10 minutes.

3. Meanwhile, in a medium bowl, combine applesauce, maple syrup, ketchup, lemon juice, cinnamon, paprika, garlic powder, Salt-Shaker Substitute, and pepper. Stir to blend.

4. Arrange spareribs in the prepared baking pan, spacing them slightly apart. Spoon ½ sauce over spareribs. Bake, uncovered, for 1½ hours or until done, basting with remaining sauce about every 20 minutes.

PINCH OF SAGE

This recipe makes plenty of barbecue sauce so you can reserve a portion to serve as a dipping sauce with the spareribs. To avoid contamination, be sure to bring the barbecue sauce to a boil before serving as you would a marinade that's been in contact with raw meat.

Spaghetti and Meatballs in Marinara Sauce

Lightly seasoned ground beef meatballs and whole-wheat spaghetti are topped with a mild, vegetable-rich tomato sauce.

Yield:	Prep time:	Cook time:	Serving size:
8 servings	10 minutes	40 minutes	2 ounces spaghetti with ½ cup sauce and 3 meatballs

Each serving has:		
455.6 calories	89 mg sodium	

¼ cup extra-virgin olive oil

3 medium yellow onions, chopped

2 medium cloves garlic, chopped

6 large baby carrots, halved and sliced

2 (14.5-oz.) cans no-salt-added diced tomatoes, with juice

1 lb. 85-percent-lean ground beef

¼ tsp. freshly ground black pepper

2½ tsp. dried oregano

2 tsp. dried basil

3 TB. unsalted butter

1 (16-oz.) pkg. whole-wheat spaghetti

1. In a large saucepan over medium heat, heat extra-virgin olive oil. Add onions, garlic, and carrots, and sauté for 6 minutes or until onions are translucent. Stir in tomatoes.

2. Transfer mixture to a food processor, and process for 45 seconds or until smooth, scraping down the sides as necessary. Return to the saucepan, and bring to a boil. Reduce heat as needed to maintain a simmer, cover, and simmer for 15 minutes.

3. Meanwhile, in a large bowl, combine ground beef, pepper, 1 teaspoon oregano, and 1 teaspoon basil until evenly distributed. Shape into 24 (1½-inch) meatballs.

4. Stir butter, remaining 1½ teaspoons oregano, and remaining 1 teaspoon basil into the saucepan. Simmer, covered, for 15 more minutes.

5. In a large nonstick skillet over medium heat, cook meatballs for 12 minutes or until done. Using a slotted spoon, remove meatballs to a paper towel–lined plate and blot dry.

6. Add meatballs to marinara sauce, and continue to simmer, covered, while spaghetti cooks.

7. Cook spaghetti according to the package directions (omit salt). Drain.

8. Serve marinara sauce and meatballs over spaghetti.

Salternative: Season the sauce with a salt-free salt substitute seasoning blend, if you prefer. You may also substitute the tomato sauce from the Individual Lasagna Casseroles recipe in Chapter 18.

PINCH OF SAGE

To save on preparation and cooking time, you can use a commercially produced no-salt-added pasta sauce instead of preparing the marinara sauce from scratch.

Just-Like-Mom's Meat Loaf

Ground beef, pork, and veal combine in a moist loaf topped with a tangy-sweet tomato sauce.

Yield:	Prep time:	Cook time:	Serving size:
7 or 8 servings	15 minutes	65 minutes	1 (1¼-inch) slice
Each serving has:			
368.3 calories	115.8 mg sodium		

½ cup no-salt-added ketchup

¼ cup firmly packed light brown sugar

4 tsp. cider vinegar

2 tsp. extra-virgin olive oil

1 medium yellow onion, diced

2 medium cloves garlic, minced

½ tsp. dried thyme

1 tsp. Salt-Shaker Substitute (recipe in Chapter 14) or other savory salt-free salt substitute seasoning blend

½ tsp. freshly ground black pepper

¼ tsp. dry mustard

¼ tsp. cayenne

2 TB. dried parsley flakes

½ cup fat-free plain yogurt

2 large eggs

1¾ to 2 lb. meat loaf mix (ground beef, ground pork, ground veal)

⅔ cup quick oats

1. In a small bowl, stir together ketchup, light brown sugar, and cider vinegar. Set glaze aside.

2. In a small skillet over medium heat, heat extra-virgin olive oil. Add onion and garlic, and sauté for 5 minutes or until tender. Set aside.

3. Preheat the oven to 350°F. Line a shallow baking pan with nonstick aluminum foil.

4. In a large bowl, combine thyme, Salt-Shaker Substitute, pepper, dry mustard, cayenne, parsley flakes, yogurt, and eggs. Stir until evenly blended.

5. Add meat loaf mix, oats, and onion mixture, and mix with your hands until thoroughly blended. Transfer to the prepared baking pan, and form into a 9×5-inch loaf. Spoon ½ glaze over top of loaf.

6. Bake for 45 minutes. Brush remaining glaze over top of loaf, and bake for 15 more minutes or until done (160°F on a food thermometer). Let stand for 15 to 20 minutes before cutting into 1¼-inch slices.

PINCH OF SAGE

If you prefer, serve the remaining glaze on the side instead of brushing it over the top of the loaf at the end of baking. To do this, pour the glaze into a small saucepan over medium-low heat, and bring it to a gentle boil. Cook, stirring, until slightly thickened, and serve with meat loaf slices.

Steak and Veggie Shish Kebabs

Simply peppered beef steak cubes are threaded with fresh vegetables and quick-broiled.

Yield:	Prep time:	Cook time:	Serving size:
8 skewers	20 minutes	10 minutes	2 skewers
Each serving has:			
243.7 calories	119.2 mg sodium		

1¼ lb. chuck beef steak, trimmed and cut into 2-in. cubes; or 1½-in. kebab cubes; or ¾-in.-thick boneless rib eye, trimmed and cut into 2-in. cubes

8 medium button mushroom caps, wiped with a damp paper towel

1 medium zucchini, cut into 8 thick slices

8 (½- to 2-in.) chunks green bell peppers

8 (½- to 2-in.) chunks yellow bell peppers

8 (½- to 2-in.-thick) chunks sweet onion

8 cherry tomatoes

1 TB. extra-virgin olive oil

¼ tsp. freshly ground black pepper

1. Preheat the broiler to high. Spray the rack of a broiler pan with nonstick cooking spray.

2. Thread beef cubes, mushroom caps, zucchini, green bell peppers, yellow bell peppers, sweet onions, and cherry tomatoes onto 8 wooden or metal skewers, spacing them slightly apart.

3. Lightly brush extra-virgin olive oil over beef, mushroom caps, zucchini, and sweet onions. Season beef with pepper.

4. Arrange skewers on the rack of the broiler pan. Broil 3 or 4 inches from the heat source for 10 minutes, turning after 5 minutes, or until beef is done as desired (160°F for medium).

PINCH OF SAGE

Serve these skewers over rice for a great meal. And when the weather's nice, prepare the shish kebabs on a hot grill—just remember to soak wooden skewers in water for at least 30 minutes first to prevent burning.

Beef Tips with Onions and Mushrooms

Tender, slow-simmered steak bites, sautéed onions, and meaty mushrooms are enveloped in a beefy sauce.

Yield:	Prep time:	Cook time:	Serving size:
4 cups	5 minutes	1 hour, 10 minutes	1 cup
Each serving has:			
326.4 calories	167.1 mg sodium		

2 TB. unsalted butter

2 TB. all-purpose flour

1 cup unsalted beef stock

½ cup Sodium-Wise Soy Sauce Stand-In (recipe in Chapter 12)

1 bay leaf

1 lb. sirloin tip steak, trimmed of all visible fat

2 tsp. extra-virgin olive oil

1 cup halved and thinly sliced yellow onions

3 cups small baby portobello mushrooms or crimini mushrooms, trimmed (halve larger mushrooms)

1 medium clove garlic, minced

½ tsp. Salt-Shaker Substitute (recipe in Chapter 14) or other salt-free salt substitute seasoning blend

¼ tsp. freshly ground black pepper

1. In a large saucepan over medium heat, melt butter. Stir in flour, and cook, stirring constantly, for 3 minutes or until bubbly, smooth, and golden brown.

2. Slowly stir in beef stock and Sodium-Wise Soy Sauce Stand-In. Add bay leaf, and bring to a simmer, reducing heat if necessary to maintain a simmer.

3. Meanwhile, heat a large, nonstick skillet over medium heat. When hot, add sirloin tip steak, and cook for 5 minutes, turning to brown on all sides. Drain well.

4. Add steak to beef stock mixture, stir, and increase heat to high, and bring to a boil. Reduce heat as needed to maintain a simmer, cover, and simmer for 45 minutes.

5. Meanwhile, in the large skillet over medium heat, heat extra-virgin olive oil for 30 seconds. Stir in onions and mushrooms, and cook for 5 minutes or until softened. Stir in garlic, and cook for 1 minute.

6. Add Salt-Shaker Substitute and pepper to beef stock mixture, and stir. Add onion mixture, and stir. Cover and simmer for 15 minutes or until steak is tender. Remove and discard bay leaf.

7. Serve over whole-wheat egg noodles or brown rice as desired.

PINCH OF SAGE

Bay leaves impart a mild citrus taste to recipes, but they're not pleasant to bite into unexpectedly. Remember to remove the sharp-edged leaf before serving—or at least warn your diners to keep an eye out if you're unable to locate it.

Slow Cooker Saucy Pork Shoulder Roast

Melt-in-your-mouth pork is ladled with a spicy reduction sauce.

Yield:	Prep time:	Cook time:	Serving size:
6 servings	8 minutes	9½ to 10½ hours	3 ounces cooked meat with sauce

Each serving has:		
347.9 calories	175 mg sodium	

½ cup water

¼ cup Southern Heat BBQ Dry Rub (recipe in Chapter 14)

1 (3- to 3½-lb.) bone-in pork shoulder blade roast

1. Pour water into the bottom of a 5-quart slow cooker, and add a steamer basket that sits above the water.

2. Work Southern Heat BBQ Dry Rub into pork roast, and set on the steamer basket in the slow cooker. Cover and cook on low heat for 9 or 10 hours or until fork-tender.

3. Remove pork roast from the slow cooker and keep warm.

4. Strain liquid into a small saucepan, and bring to a boil over high heat. Reduce heat to medium to medium-low, and boil gently for 30 minutes or until liquid is slightly thickened and reduced to about $\frac{2}{3}$ cup, stirring and watching carefully to prevent boiling over.

5. To serve, remove bone (it should pull out easily) and trim fat well. Slice pork roast, and pour reduction over top.

PINCH OF SAGE

After you've poured the liquid from the slow cooker, you can return the pork roast to the turned-off slow cooker and cover to keep it warm.

Cincinnati Chili–Style Dinner

Chunky two-bean and beef chili tops whole-wheat capellini sprinkled with melty cheddar cheese.

Yield:	Prep time:	Cook time:	Serving size:
7 servings	10 minutes	1 hour, 40 minutes	2 ounces pasta with 1 cup chili

Each serving has:	
580.7 calories	218.9 mg sodium

¾ lb. 85-percent-lean ground beef

2 medium yellow onions, chopped

1 medium green bell pepper, ribs and seeds removed, and chopped

1 (14.5-oz.) can no-salt-added diced tomatoes, with juice

1 (15-oz.) can no-salt-added tomato sauce

1 (15-oz.) can no-salt-added small red beans, rinsed and drained

1 (15-oz.) can no-salt-added cannellini beans (white kidney beans), rinsed and drained

2½ tsp. Firehouse Chili Powder (recipe in Chapter 14) or other salt-free chili powder

1½ tsp. Salt-Shaker Substitute (recipe in Chapter 14) or other salt-free salt substitute seasoning blend

¼ tsp. paprika

¼ tsp. ground ginger

14 oz. whole-wheat capellini

1 cup shredded low-sodium cheddar cheese

1. In a large saucepan over medium heat, brown ground beef with 1 chopped onion and green bell pepper for 7 minutes or until meat is browned and onions are translucent. Drain well.

2. Add diced tomatoes, tomato sauce, red beans, and cannellini beans, and stir. Add Firehouse Chili Powder, Salt-Shaker Substitute, paprika, and ginger, and stir. Bring to a boil. Reduce heat as needed to maintain a simmer, cover, and simmer for 1½ hours.

3. Meanwhile, about 10 minutes before saucepan mixture is done simmering, cook capellini according to the package directions (omit salt). Drain.

4. To assemble, line each of 7 plates with capellini. Ladle on chili, and scatter cheddar cheese and remaining chopped onion on top.

PINCH OF SAGE

For a quick-fix dinner, prepare the chili the night before and heat it up the next day.

Versatile Vegetable Mains

In This Chapter

- Filling your plate with vegetables and grains
- Stretching your budget with meatless entrées
- Filling up on fiber
- Serving cholesterol-free dishes

When you want something hearty, fresh, and delicious for dinner, consider a meatless meal. Just because you aren't serving meat doesn't mean you're giving up flavor; vegetables provide plenty of great tastes. Plus, flavorful vegetables and whole grains supply fiber, which slows digestion and helps you feel full and satisfied.

If your dietary needs include low-cholesterol meals, meatless meals make it easy. Many of the recipes included in this chapter are cholesterol free, and you can omit the cheese in the others.

What's more, most vegetables, pastas, grains, herbs, and spices are reasonably priced. Great taste, low cost, high fiber, low cholesterol—it's win-win again and again!

Fresh Food for Less

You'll see one of the benefits of preparing a meatless main dish every now and then when you look at your grocery receipt. Fresh vegetables and grains are comfortably affordable. And if you're a gardener, you may have a bumper crop of any of these ingredients you'll want to use at their peak of freshness.

Even if you don't have a garden full of veggies to pick from, the dishes in this chapter give you a great excuse to comb local farmers' markets and roadside stands for the freshest produce at the best price. Nothing beats the taste of freshly picked veggies, and after a few meals, you may have your family asking especially for these dishes!

Here's to Your Health!

Vegetables and whole grains naturally provide plenty of fiber. A main dish made of these ingredients helps you reach the 25 (or more) grams requirement you should meet each day. If you need to boost your fiber intake, try substituting a whole-wheat pasta or grain in any recipe.

Additionally, eating a meatless meal often enables you to choose a cholesterol-free dinner. Cholesterol—it's bad, it's good, it's confusing. Cholesterol is a waxy-type substance transported through your blood by lipoproteins. *Low-density lipoprotein* (*LDL*) can contribute to plaque buildup in your arteries—this is "bad" cholesterol. *High-density lipoprotein* (*HDL*) moves cholesterol from the arteries to the liver to be passed out of your body—this is the "good" cholesterol.

> **DEFINITION**
>
> **Low-density lipoprotein** (**LDL**) carries cholesterol through your arteries contributing to arterial plaque—hard deposits that may block the arteries. Reduce your risk of heart attack or stroke by keeping your LDL below 160 mg/dL (below 100, if you have heart disease). **High-density lipoprotein** (**HDL**) moves cholesterol to your liver to be passed from your body. HDL may even take cholesterol out of plaques, slowing development. You want an HDL number of 40 mg/dL (50 mg/dL for women) or above.

Your body produces cholesterol, and you also ingest cholesterol from animal sources such as meats, poultry, fish and seafood, whole dairy products, and eggs. By choosing a meatless meal (hold the cheese), you can keep your cholesterol intake to a minimum. You'll find several heart-healthy meals in this chapter to get you started.

Moroccan Couscous-Stuffed Peppers

Tart and savory sun-dried tomatoes play against smooth and sweet pine nuts and raisins in couscous-stuffed bell peppers with a touch of cinnamon.

Yield:	Prep time:	Cook time:	Serving size:
2 bell pepper halves	10 minutes	30 minutes	1 bell pepper half

Each serving has:			
243.3 calories	1 mg sodium		

3 TB. unsalted pine nuts

½ tsp. extra-virgin olive oil

1 small yellow onion, diced

1 medium clove garlic, minced

¾ cup cooked whole-wheat couscous or regular couscous

4 dry-packed sun-dried tomatoes, rehydrated and chopped

3 TB. golden raisins

⅛ tsp. freshly ground black pepper

Large pinch ground cinnamon

1 large red, yellow, or orange bell pepper, ribs and seeds removed, and halved

1. Preheat the oven to 375°F. Spray a small baking dish with nonstick cooking spray.

2. In a small skillet over medium heat, toast pine nuts for 3 minutes or until golden, shaking occasionally to keep from burning. Remove pine nuts to a small bowl.

3. Add extra-virgin olive oil to the skillet. Add onion, and sauté for 2 minutes or until softened and lightly golden. Add garlic, and sauté for 30 seconds.

4. Add onion and garlic to the bowl with pine nuts. Stir in couscous, sun-dried tomatoes, golden raisins, pepper, and cinnamon. Blend well.

5. Spoon mixture into bell pepper halves, and place peppers in the prepared dish. Bake for 20 minutes or until golden brown on top and bell peppers are tender-crisp.

 SALT PITFALL

Opt for dry-packed sun-dried tomatoes found in plastic packaging. The jarred type packed in olive oil are processed with sodium.

Herbed Red Bell Pepper Sauce over Vermicelli

Rosemary brightens the red bell pepper and balsamic vinegar purée that coats this pasta.

Yield:	Prep time:	Cook time:	Serving size:
4 servings	10 minutes	10 minutes	2 ounces pasta with ½ cup sauce

Each serving has:	
291.3 calories	11.6 mg sodium

8 oz. vermicelli pasta

2 medium red bell peppers, ribs and seeds removed, and chopped

¼ cup balsamic vinegar

2 TB. extra-virgin olive oil

3 medium cloves garlic, minced

2 TB. chopped fresh rosemary leaves

1 TB. chopped fresh oregano leaves

½ tsp. crushed red pepper flakes

½ cup chopped fresh parsley

1. Cook pasta according to the package directions (omit salt). Drain.

2. In a food processor, process red bell peppers with balsamic vinegar until very finely chopped.

3. In a small saucepan over medium-low heat, heat extra-virgin olive oil. Add garlic, and sauté for 1 or 2 minutes or until golden. Stir in rosemary, oregano, and crushed red pepper flakes.

4. Add red bell pepper mixture, and stir to combine. Increase heat to medium, and bring to a simmer. Remove from heat, stir in parsley, and spoon sauce over pasta to serve.

Salternative: This sauce is also good over other pasta shapes, such as rotini, bow ties, or pipette.

 PINCH OF SAGE

Kitchen shears make quick work of chopping fresh herbs. You can keep the blades sharp by cutting through a piece of steel wool occasionally.

Bell Pepper Pasta Sauce over Capellini

Tender bell pepper and onion slices, fresh plum tomatoes, and a touch of heat top whole-wheat pasta.

Yield:	Prep time:	Cook time:	Serving size:
4 servings	10 minutes	20 minutes	2 ounces pasta with ½ cup sauce

Each serving has:	
333.8 calories	20.2 mg sodium

3 TB. extra-virgin olive oil

1 cup thinly sliced green, red, and yellow bell peppers

1 medium yellow onion, halved and thinly sliced

2 large cloves garlic, minced

1½ lb. plum tomatoes (about 10 or 11), cored and diced

8 oz. whole-wheat capellini pasta or thin spaghetti

½ tsp. crushed red pepper flakes

Pinch freshly ground black pepper

1 TB. finely chopped fresh basil or more to taste

1. In a large, heavy skillet over medium heat, heat 1 tablespoon extra-virgin olive oil. Add bell peppers and onion, and sauté for 5 or 6 minutes or until tender (without browning), stirring frequently.

2. Add garlic and tomatoes, and stir. Increase heat to medium-high, and cook for 13 to 15 minutes or until thickened.

3. Meanwhile, cook pasta according to the package directions (omit salt). Drain.

4. Remove the skillet from heat. Stir in crushed red pepper flakes, pepper, and basil. Stir in remaining 2 tablespoons olive oil, and serve sauce over pasta.

Salternative: Add a dash of salt-free salt substitute seasoning blend when you add the black pepper, if you prefer. You also may substitute dried basil for fresh by using 1 teaspoon dried basil or more to taste.

PINCH OF SAGE

Plum, Roma, Italian, Saladette, egg, processing, paste, or sauce tomatoes? No matter what name you call these small, oval tomatoes, you'll enjoy their flavorful, meaty flesh that's great for making sauces.

Winter Vegetable Spaghetti

Heady cauliflower and broccoli florets join flavorful sautéed onions in a seasoned olive oil sauce tossed with thin spaghetti.

Yield:	Prep time:	Cook time:	Serving size:
12 cups	10 minutes	15 minutes	2 cups

Each serving has:	
389.7 calories	36.9 mg sodium

1 (13.25-oz.) pkg. whole-wheat thin spaghetti	1 medium yellow onion, diced
½ medium head cauliflower, broken into small florets	2 medium cloves garlic, minced
	3 TB. chopped fresh parsley, or 1 tsp. dried parsley flakes
2 medium stalks broccoli, broken into small florets	¼ tsp. garlic powder
7 TB. extra-virgin olive oil	¼ tsp. freshly ground black pepper

1. Cook spaghetti according to the package directions (omit salt). Drain.

2. Meanwhile, fill a steamer pot or a large saucepan with enough water to fall below the steamer basket when added, and bring to a boil over high heat. Add cauliflower and broccoli to a steamer basket, and place the basket in the pot or saucepan. Cover and steam vegetables over gently boiling water, reducing heat as necessary, for 5 to 7 minutes or until fork-tender.

3. In a large skillet over medium-low to medium heat, heat extra-virgin olive oil. Add onion and garlic, and sauté for 5 minutes or until tender and lightly golden.

4. Stir in parsley, garlic powder, and pepper, and sauté for 1 minute. Stir in cauliflower and broccoli.

5. In a large serving bowl, toss spaghetti with cauliflower mixture, and serve.

SALT PITFALL

When cooking spaghetti, remember to omit the optional salt from the cooking water. Omit any optional oil as well to keep from adding unnecessary fat to your dish. Just remember to stir the spaghetti occasionally to keep it from clumping or sticking.

Fresh Tomato and Mozzarella Ziti

Pasta, creamy mozzarella, and garden-fresh tomatoes are Italian-seasoned and spiced with hot red pepper flakes.

Yield:	Prep time:	Cook time:	Serving size:
6 cups	10 minutes	10 minutes	1½ cups
Each serving has:			
419.1 calories	50.6 mg sodium		

¼ cup extra-virgin olive oil

¼ cup chopped fresh basil

1 TB. chopped fresh oregano

¼ tsp. crushed red pepper flakes

2 medium cloves garlic, minced

¼ tsp. freshly ground black pepper

4 oz. fresh mozzarella cheese, coarsely chopped

2 large tomatoes, cored and diced

8 oz. ziti pasta

1. In a large serving bowl, combine extra-virgin olive oil, basil, oregano, crushed red pepper flakes, garlic, pepper, mozzarella cheese, and tomatoes. Set aside to allow flavors to mingle and mixture to reach room temperature.

2. Meanwhile, cook pasta according to the package directions (omit salt). Drain well, and add to the serving bowl. Stir to combine, and serve immediately.

Salternative: Serve this no-cook sauce with other pasta shapes, such as penne, bow ties, or linguini.

SALT PITFALL

Be sure to choose fresh mozzarella cheese, which is naturally lower in sodium. The lowest-sodium fresh mozzarella is usually sold packed in water, but, of course, read those labels.

Tofu and Veggie Stir-Fry

Spicy, sweet orange sauce flavors crisp-tender Asian-style veggies and silky tofu cubes.

Yield:	Prep time:	Cook time:	Serving size:
4 servings	10 minutes	6 minutes	1 cup stir-fry with $\frac{1}{2}$ cup rice

Each serving has:	
276 calories	51.8 mg sodium

2 TB. sesame oil

2 medium cloves garlic, minced

$\frac{1}{2}$ tsp. ground ginger

1 cup julienned zucchini

1 cup julienned yellow squash

1 cup sliced button mushrooms

$\frac{1}{2}$ medium red bell pepper, ribs and seeds removed, and cut into thin strips

$\frac{1}{2}$ cup Chinese snow peas, trimmed

1 (16-oz.) pkg. firm tofu, drained, squeezed, and cut into cubes

$\frac{1}{2}$ tsp. cayenne

$\frac{1}{2}$ tsp. onion powder

$\frac{1}{2}$ tsp. cornstarch

$\frac{1}{4}$ cup unsweetened orange juice

2 cups cooked long-grain brown rice

1. In a wok or a large skillet over medium-high heat, heat sesame oil, garlic, and ginger. When sizzling, add zucchini, yellow squash, mushrooms, red bell pepper, and snow peas. Cook, stirring, for 2 minutes.

2. Add tofu, cayenne, and onion powder, and cook, stirring, for 2 or 3 minutes.

3. In a small bowl, stir cornstarch into orange juice. Pour into wok, and cook, stirring, for 1 minute. Remove the wok from heat, and serve tofu and veggies over rice.

PINCH OF SAGE

The secret to stir-frying is to have all your ingredients ready. Once you start cooking, you have to keep stirring. But in the end, you'll have a nutrition-packed meal ready in no time.

Grilled Veggie Pasta Toss

Smoky, sizzled vegetables top pasta with a slightly sweet, herbed balsamic sauce.

Yield:	Prep time:	Cook time:	Serving size:
6 servings	5 minutes	10 minutes	2 ounces pasta with 1 cup veggies

Each serving has:	
262.9 calories	57.1 mg sodium

12 oz. bow-tie pasta

6 cups Hearty Grilled Veggie Salad (recipe in Chapter 5), warmed

¾ cup coarsely shredded fresh mozzarella cheese

1. Cook pasta according to the package directions (omit salt). Drain.

2. To serve, line 6 plates with pasta. Spoon warm Hearty Grilled Veggie Salad over pasta. Sprinkle 2 tablespoons mozzarella cheese over each serving.

PINCH OF SAGE

Should you have any leftover Hearty Grilled Veggie Salad, this recipe is a great way to enjoy those leftovers. Cook enough pasta and shred enough cheese for the amount of vegetables you have remaining.

Garden-Fresh Balsamic Tomato Sauce over Angel Hair

Summer-picked tomatoes and basil meld their flavors with sweet balsamic vinegar in this pleasant no-cook sauce for pasta.

Yield:	Prep time:	Cook time:	Serving size:
6 servings	10 minutes	5 minutes	2 ounces pasta with 1 cup sauce

Each serving has:	
321.6 calories	87.7 mg sodium

5 cups diced tomatoes, cored	2 TB. extra-virgin olive oil
1 cup diced yellow onions	1 tsp. granulated sugar
3 medium cloves garlic, minced	12 oz. whole-wheat angel hair pasta
½ cup chopped fresh basil, or 2½ TB. dried basil	¾ cup coarsely shredded fresh mozzarella cheese
¼ cup balsamic vinegar	

1. In a large, *nonreactive* bowl, combine tomatoes, onions, garlic, basil, balsamic vinegar, extra-virgin olive oil, and sugar. Stir well, and cover with plastic wrap. Let stand at room temperature for at least 3 or 4 hours.

2. Cook pasta according to the package directions (omit salt). Drain.

3. To serve, line plates with pasta, top with sauce, and sprinkle 2 tablespoons mozzarella cheese on each serving.

Salternative: If you're trying to save on your sodium count, this dish is just as good without the mozzarella cheese.

DEFINITION

When a recipe calls for a **nonreactive** dish, use glass, stainless steel, enameled ceramic, or other material. These won't react with the acid in the tomatoes and vinegar as an aluminum or copper bowl would.

Southwestern-Style Quinoa-Stuffed Peppers

Mild, whole-grain *quinoa* is spiced up with cilantro, cumin, black beans, and sweet corn in flavorful bell pepper halves.

Yield:	Prep time:	Cook time:	Serving size:
4 bell pepper halves	5 minutes	45 minutes	1 bell pepper half

Each serving has:		
222 calories	125.1 mg sodium	

2 tsp. extra-virgin olive oil

$\frac{1}{2}$ cup diced yellow onions

2 medium cloves garlic, minced

$\frac{1}{2}$ cup uncooked quinoa

1 cup reduced-sodium fat-free chicken broth or vegetable broth

$\frac{1}{2}$ tsp. ground cumin

$\frac{1}{4}$ tsp. cayenne

$\frac{1}{8}$ tsp. Salt-Shaker Substitute (recipe in Chapter 14) or other salt-free salt substitute seasoning blend

1 cup cooked black beans, drained

$\frac{2}{3}$ cup frozen whole-kernel corn

$\frac{1}{4}$ cup chopped fresh cilantro

2 large green or red bell peppers, ribs and seeds removed, and halved

Boiling water as needed

1. Heat a medium saucepan over medium-low heat. When hot, add extra-virgin olive oil, and heat for 1 minute. Add onions, and cook for 5 minutes or until softened, stirring occasionally.

2. Add garlic, and cook, stirring, for 1 minute. Add quinoa, and cook for 1 minute.

3. Slowly add chicken broth. Add cumin, cayenne, and Salt-Shaker Substitute, and stir. Increase heat to high, and bring to a boil. Reduce heat to low, cover, and simmer for 15 to 20 minutes or until liquid is just absorbed.

4. Preheat the oven to 400°F.

5. Turn off heat. Stir in black beans, corn, and cilantro. Spoon into bell pepper halves.

6. Arrange stuffed bell pepper halves in a 2-quart casserole dish or other dish large enough to hold stuffed peppers in a single layer. Pour in enough boiling water to cover the bottom of the dish $\frac{1}{2}$ inch deep. Cover and bake for 20 minutes or until bell peppers are fork-tender. Carefully remove stuffed peppers with a slotted spoon to serve.

DEFINITION

Quinoa is a mild whole grain that's been rinsed of a naturally occurring, bitter-tasting residue. Check your package to be certain the grains have been prewashed. If not, rinse and drain the quinoa before cooking.

Chunky Tomato Sauce and Kidney Beans over Spaghetti Squash

Savory sautéed vegetables and kidney beans are flavored with fresh herbs and served over sweet strands of winter squash.

Yield:	Prep time:	Cook time:	Serving size:
4 cups squash and 4 cups sauce	25 minutes	1 hour	1 cup squash and 1 cup sauce

Each serving has:	
275.8 calories	133.1 mg sodium

1 small (about 2 lb.) *spaghetti squash*

2 tsp. extra-virgin olive oil

1 cup coarsely chopped red onions

1 cup coarsely chopped green bell peppers

1 cup sliced button mushrooms

2 medium cloves garlic, minced

¼ tsp. crushed red pepper flakes

2 cups coarsely chopped tomatoes

2 TB. chopped fresh basil

2 TB. chopped fresh Italian parsley

1 (16-oz.) can reduced-sodium dark red kidney beans, rinsed and drained

1. Preheat the oven to 375°F.

2. Prick whole spaghetti squash with a skewer all over. Place spaghetti squash in a baking dish large enough to hold squash comfortably. Bake for 1 hour. Let stand for 20 minutes or until cool enough to handle.

3. Meanwhile, heat a large nonstick skillet over medium-low to medium heat. Add extra-virgin olive oil, and heat for 1 minute. Add red onions, green bell peppers, and mushrooms, and cook, stirring occasionally, for 8 minutes or until softened.

4. Add garlic and crushed red pepper flakes, and cook, stirring frequently, for 2 minutes. Add tomatoes, basil, and Italian parsley. Cook, stirring occasionally, for 3 minutes or until tomatoes have released their liquid. Add kidney beans and cook, stirring occasionally, for 2 minutes or until heated through.

5. Cut spaghetti squash in half lengthwise. Using a spoon, scrape out and discard seeds. Using a fork, scrape out squash flesh in strands.

6. To serve, line serving plates with spaghetti squash and spoon bean mixture over top.

DEFINITION

Spaghetti squash is a yellow-skinned winter squash that gets its name because its baked flesh releases from its shell in long, spaghetti-like strands when scraped loose with a fork. This squash makes a good substitute for the pasta as well.

Veggie-Topped Polenta Pizza Squares

Seasoned tomato sauce, cheese, and classic vegetable toppings add pizza-style flavor to a mild, thick *polenta* crust.

Yield:	Prep time:	Cook time:	Serving size:
8 slices	15 minutes	20 minutes	2 slices
Each serving has:			
374.3 calories	189.6 mg sodium		

5 cups hot, cooked polenta

1 (8-oz.) can no-salt-added tomato sauce

¼ tsp. dried basil

⅛ tsp. dried oregano

⅛ tsp. garlic powder

⅛ tsp. onion powder

⅛ tsp. freshly ground black pepper

1 cup coarsely shredded fresh mozzarella cheese

1 small tomato, thinly sliced

½ small yellow onion, sliced

¼ medium green bell pepper, ribs and seeds removed, and thinly sliced

2 medium button mushrooms, wiped with a damp paper towel and sliced

2 TB. sliced black olives or no-salt-added sliced black olives

1. Preheat the oven to 350°F. Spray a 13×9×2-inch baking dish with nonstick cooking spray.

2. Spoon polenta into the prepared baking dish, forming a crust with a rim around the edges.

3. In a small bowl, stir together tomato sauce, basil, oregano, garlic powder, onion powder, and pepper.

4. Spoon tomato sauce mixture over crust. Sprinkle on mozzarella cheese, and top with tomato slices, onion slices, green bell pepper slices, mushroom slices, and olive slices. Bake for 20 minutes or until hot and cheese is bubbly. Let stand for 5 minutes before cutting and serving with a fork.

Salternative: If you prefer a thinner crust, use a little less polenta.

> **DEFINITION**
>
> **Polenta** is cornmeal mush. Prepare it according to the package directions, omitting the salt as you would when preparing pasta, noodles, rice, and hot cooked cereals.

Quinoa with Wilted Greens and Beans

Heady kale, creamy white beans, and crunchy walnuts enliven mild, whole-grain quinoa.

Yield:	Prep time:	Cook time:	Serving size:
7½ cups	5 minutes	30 minutes	1¼ cups
Each serving has:			
317.8 calories	188.2 mg sodium		

3 tsp. extra-virgin olive oil

½ cup diced yellow onions

2 medium cloves garlic, minced

1 cup uncooked quinoa

2 cups reduced-sodium fat-free chicken broth or vegetable broth

4 cups packed torn kale, large stems removed

½ cup water

1 TB. fresh lemon juice

¼ tsp. crushed red pepper flakes

2 cups cooked Great Northern beans, drained

½ cup coarsely chopped unsalted walnuts

1. Heat a medium saucepan over medium heat. Add 1 teaspoon extra-virgin olive oil, and heat for 30 seconds. Add onions, and cook for 2 minutes or until golden, stirring frequently.

2. Add garlic, and cook for 1 minute, stirring frequently. Add quinoa, and cook for 2 minutes or until golden, stirring frequently.

3. Slowly pour chicken broth into quinoa mixture. Bring to a boil, cover, reduce heat to low, and simmer for 15 minutes or until liquid is absorbed.

4. Meanwhile, in an extra-large nonstick skillet over medium heat, combine kale and water. Cook, stirring occasionally, for 15 minutes or until wilted and skillet is dry.

5. Stir remaining 2 teaspoons extra-virgin olive oil, lemon juice, and crushed red pepper flakes into kale. Add Great Northern beans and walnuts, and cook for 3 minutes or until walnuts are fragrant, stirring occasionally.

6. Add quinoa mixture, and cook, stirring, for 1 or 2 more minutes or until combined and heated through.

SALT PITFALL

Kale's tight, crinkled leaves tend to trap sand and dirt. Wash kale leaves very well just before using.

Acorn Squash Stuffed with Cranberry-Nut Wild Rice

This wild rice medley subtly flavored with fruits and nuts is enhanced by the velvety sweetness of acorn squash.

Yield:	Prep time:	Cook time:	Serving size:
2 squash halves	8 minutes	1½ hours	1 squash half
Each serving has:			
460.5 calories	357.1 mg sodium		

¼ cup chopped unsalted walnuts

½ cup uncooked wild rice

1½ cups reduced-sodium fat-free chicken broth or vegetable broth

¼ tsp. onion powder

¼ cup dried cranberries

1 medium acorn squash

1. In a medium saucepan over medium heat, toast walnuts for 2 minutes or until fragrant, shaking the saucepan occasionally to prevent burning.

2. Stir in wild rice, and toast for 3 minutes or until toasted, stirring occasionally.

3. Slowly pour in chicken broth, stir in onion powder, and stir in dried cranberries. Increase heat to high, and bring to a boil. Reduce heat to low, cover, and simmer for 1 hour, 10 minutes, or until most of liquid has been absorbed. Remove from heat, uncover, stir, and let stand for 5 minutes.

4. Toward the end of the rice mixture cook time, preheat the oven to 375°F.

5. Carefully cut squash in half lengthwise. Using a spoon, scoop out and discard seeds. Arrange squash halves cut side down in a 9×9×2 baking dish or other dish large enough to hold squash comfortably and fill the dish with $\frac{1}{2}$ inch water. Bake for 30 minutes or until squash is just fork-tender.

6. Remove the casserole dish from the oven. Remove squash halves, and drain water from the dish. Return squash halves to the dish cut side up. Spoon wild rice mixture evenly into hollows of squash halves. Bake for 15 minutes or until squash is tender and rice has absorbed broth.

PINCH OF SAGE

Thick-skinned winter squash such as acorn can be stored whole in a cool, dark place for 2 months.

Individual Lasagna Casseroles

Tasty zucchini slices add their flavor to the traditional layering of pasta, cheese, and tomatoes.

Yield:	Prep time:	Cook time:	Serving size:
4 casseroles	20 minutes	40 minutes	1 casserole

Each serving has:			
529.5 calories	386 mg sodium		

6 lasagna noodles

2 TB. extra-virgin olive oil

2 medium cloves garlic, minced

1 (15-oz.) can no-salt-added tomato sauce

1 (14.5-oz.) can no-salt-added diced tomatoes, with juice

1 tsp. dried basil

½ tsp. dried oregano

1 tsp. Salt-Shaker Substitute (recipe in Chapter 14)

1 tsp. freshly ground black pepper

1¾ cups coarsely shredded fresh mozzarella cheese

1 cup light ricotta cheese

1 large egg

8 (⅛- to ¼-in.-thick) lengthwise slices medium zucchini

1. Cook lasagna noodles according to the package directions (omit salt). Drain and cut in half.

2. In a medium saucepan over medium heat, heat extra-virgin olive oil. Add garlic, and sauté for 30 seconds or until garlic sizzles.

3. Add tomato sauce, diced tomatoes, basil, oregano, Salt-Shaker Substitute, and ½ teaspoon pepper. Bring to a simmer, reduce heat as needed to maintain a simmer, and simmer for 10 minutes or until slightly thickened.

4. Preheat the oven to 400°F. Place a baking sheet on the bottom oven rack in case of drips.

5. In a medium bowl, combine 1½ cups mozzarella cheese, ricotta cheese, egg, and remaining ½ teaspoon pepper. Stir until blended.

6. In 4 individual casserole serving dishes, spoon a smooth portion of sauce to cover the bottoms of the casserole dishes. Layer lasagna noodle half over sauce. Layer sauce, ½ zucchini slices, and ½ cheese mixture over top. Repeat layering. Top with noodle halves. Spoon sauce over top to cover, and sprinkle with remaining ¼ cup mozzarella cheese.

7. Bake on the top rack over baking sheet for 20 to 25 minutes or until bubbly and tender. (Tent the dishes with aluminum foil if lasagna browns too quickly.) Let stand for 5 minutes before serving.

Salternative: To save the time of preparing the sauce, substitute a commercially prepared no-salt-added pasta sauce.

PINCH OF SAGE

You can prepare this tomato sauce to use with other pasta dishes, such as the Spaghetti and Meatballs in Marinara Sauce (recipe in Chapter 17). Or use leftover sauce as a dip for the Pan-Fried Zucchini Rounds (recipe in Chapter 11).

Side by Side

At most meals, we tend to focus on the entrée. But without the wonderful foods served on the side, eating just wouldn't be as pleasurable.

You can prepare breads, salads, and side dishes—all the flavorful foods that round out our meals—with your sodium requirements in mind. Plus, you'll benefit from their contribution of fiber, vitamins, minerals, and antioxidants to your diet.

With all the great recipes in the following chapters, you're sure to find just the right accompaniments to your best main dishes.

The Bread Basket

In This Chapter

- Substituting for high-sodium leavening agents
- Working with active dry yeast
- Kneading a smooth, elastic dough
- Whipping up a quick-bread batter

Bread—it's the staff of life, traditionally made with the salt of the earth. But take heart! You can bake the comforting, homey breads you love without all the salt.

Whether you yearn for a delicious, yeasty-smelling bread or a quick-made bread, you can bake it without salt or the salty leavening agents they often require. So warm up your oven, and get ready to delight in the tempting aromas of freshly baked breads.

Sodium Switcheroo

Most bread baking requires leavening. Yeast breads use, of course, yeast to get their rise. All other breads that need a lift use baking powder and/or baking soda. Because you're reducing the sodium in your cooking, these ingredients won't fit your needs.

So to make these breads, you need to do a sodium switcheroo. Opt for sodium-free baking powder and sodium-free baking soda. These allow you to bake without all the added sodium.

When baking with sodium-free baking substitutions, read the package directions carefully because you may be required to use more (about double) the amount called for in the ingredient lists. (For more detailed information about sodium-free leavening agents, see Chapter 2.)

> **SALT PITFALL**
>
> If you start craving fresh baked goods and think a recipe is okay because it calls for just a little baking soda or baking powder, keep in mind that these leavening agents are very high in sodium. Just 1 teaspoon baking soda has 1,231 milligrams sodium. A single teaspoon of your standard double-acting aluminum sulfate baking powder contains nearly 480 milligrams sodium.

The *Yeast* You Knead to Know

The recipes in this chapter call for active dry yeast. You can purchase .25-ounce packages that contain $2\frac{1}{4}$ teaspoons yeast. Packages may also be available in larger sizes. Newer active dry yeast options include specialty yeasts for baking with whole grains. Regardless of type or size, always check the expiration date on each package because old yeast won't facilitate rising.

If a recipe requires you to dissolve the yeast in warm water or other liquid, heat the water to 100°F to 110°F. When a recipe indicates that you should combine the yeast with the flour or other dry ingredients, the added liquids should reach temperatures between 120°F to 130°F first. The best way to gauge the temperature of liquids added to yeast is to use a thermometer. If you're an old pro, you may be able to judge it by feel, but a thermometer is a bit more precise. If you get the liquids too hot, you'll kill the yeast and the bread won't rise.

When you've mixed the dough and it's time to let it rise, cover the dough in the mixing bowl or in another greased bowl with a clean dishcloth. Then, set the covered dough in a warm place to rise; the temperature should be about 80°F to 85°F. If there isn't anyplace in your home that's at least 80°F, place the covered dough on a wire rack over a pan of very hot water. You may also try placing the covered dough inside your oven with the oven light on. (Leave enough space between racks or to the broiler element for the dough to rise.) If the recipe requires a second rising, use the same methods.

Some yeast bread recipes require you to knead the dough. To do this, turn out the dough onto a lightly floured work surface. With the heels of your hands, push the dough down and forward and fold the dough over on itself, pushing it down and forward again. Give it a quarter turn, and repeat the process until the dough is smooth and elastic.

When a recipe calls for letting the dough rest, don't feel tempted to skip this step. The gluten needs to relax to achieve a desirable texture.

The Quick and the Bread

If you're not using yeast in your bread, you're making a quick bread. Contrary to the name, most quick breads take about an hour to bake. These types of breads use the term *quick* because the batter mixes up much more quickly than the process of kneading and twice rising a dough for the typical yeast bread.

Quick breads can be both sweet and savory. And you can almost always use the batters for baking muffins as well—just adjust the baking time because muffins bake much more quickly.

PINCH OF SAGE

To test if a quick bread is done, insert a cake tester or a wooden pick into the center of the loaf. If the tester comes out clean, the bread is done. If the bread is still moist inside, the tester will come out tacky with wet crumbs. If you don't have a cake tester, a strand of dry spaghetti makes a good substitute.

Fresh Tortillas

Slightly nutty thanks to its whole-wheat flour content, and lightly seasoned, this flatbread proves versatile.

Yield:	Prep time:	Cook time:	Serving size:
6 tortillas	40 minutes	15 minutes	1 tortilla

Each serving has:			
266.2 calories	0.4 mg sodium		

1 cup all-purpose flour

1 cup whole-wheat flour

2 tsp. Salt-Shaker Substitute (recipe in Chapter 14)

6 TB. trans-fat-free vegetable shortening

1 cup cool water or as needed

1. In a medium bowl, stir together all-purpose flour, whole-wheat flour, and Salt-Shaker Substitute.

2. Using a pastry blender, cut in shortening until mixture resembles coarse crumbs and no large lumps remain. Using a fork, stir in a little water at a time until dough forms a ball and cleans the bowl.

3. Turn out dough onto a well-floured work surface. Divide dough into 6 equal portions, and roll each into a ball. Cover dough with a clean dishcloth, and let rest for 15 minutes.

4. Flour a work surface, rolling pin, and your hands. Flatten each ball of dough into a circle with the heel of your hand, and roll out dough to a thin, 9- or 10-inch circle.

5. Heat a large, nonstick skillet over medium-high to medium heat. Carefully transfer dough to the skillet. Cook for 1 or 2 minutes or until done on underside. (Flatten out air bubbles a bit to ensure even cooking.) Turn and cook on the other side for 30 to 60 seconds or until browned.

PINCH OF SAGE

This recipe makes large, burrito-style tortillas. If you'd like smaller tortillas, divide the dough into 8 or 10 balls. Flatten each ball of dough with the heel of your hand and roll out the dough to a thin circle 6 to 8 inches in diameter.

Pita Pockets

These puffed up, thin white loaves are perfect for stuffing with your favorite fillings.

Yield:	Prep time:	Rise time:	Cook time:	Serving size:
8 pita pockets	1 hour, 10 minutes	1 hour	5 minutes	1 pita pocket
Each serving has:				
183.4 calories	0.6 mg sodium			

1 tsp. active dry yeast

1 cup lukewarm water (100°F to 110°F)

1 tsp. granulated sugar

1 TB. extra-light olive oil

3 cups unbleached all-purpose flour

1. In a medium bowl, dissolve yeast in lukewarm water. Stir in sugar and extra-light olive oil, and work in flour with a wooden spoon until incorporated.

2. Turn out dough onto a lightly floured work surface. Knead for 8 to 10 minutes or until perfectly smooth and elastic. Transfer dough to a large bowl sprayed with nonstick cooking spray, turning dough over to coat. Cover with a clean dishcloth, and set in a warm place to rise for 1 hour.

3. Turn out dough onto a lightly floured work surface, and gently punch down. Divide dough into 8 equal pieces, forming into balls. Cover with plastic wrap coated with nonstick cooking spray, and let rest for 10 minutes.

4. Preheat the oven to 450°F. Place 2 large baking sheets in the preheating oven.

5. Flatten each dough ball, and roll out to 6-inch circles about ¼ inch thick. Lightly sprinkle a little flour over tops, if needed. Cover with plastic wrap coated with nonstick cooking spray, and let rest for 10 minutes.

6. Transfer dough to hot baking sheets, and bake for 5 to 7 minutes or until puffed up and golden. Cool slightly on baking sheets on wire racks before serving.

PINCH OF SAGE

These pita pockets are easiest to use if you cut them in half with a sharp knife. If any didn't puff well, use the knife to slice the pocket fully open.

Mini Wheat Pita Pockets

You can tear up these small, nutty, whole-wheat puffed loaves to scoop up hummus or pack them with sandwich fixings.

Yield:	Prep time:	Rise time:	Cook time:	Serving size:
6 mini pita pockets	25 minutes	1 hour, 20 minutes	7 minutes	1 mini pita pocket
Each serving has:				
122.2 calories	2 mg sodium			

1 tsp. active dry yeast for whole grains

½ cup lukewarm water (100°F to 110°F)

½ tsp. granulated sugar

½ TB. extra-virgin olive oil

1½ cups whole-wheat flour

1. In a medium bowl, dissolve yeast in lukewarm water. Stir in sugar and extra-virgin olive oil. Work in flour with a wooden spoon to incorporate as much as possible (about 1¼ cups) to produce a cohesive dough ball.

2. Turn out dough onto a lightly floured work surface, using remaining whole-wheat flour as necessary. Knead for 8 to 10 minutes or until smooth and elastic, flouring your work surface as needed. Work dough into a ball and transfer to a medium bowl sprayed with nonstick cooking spray, turning dough over to coat. Cover with a clean dishcloth, and set in a warm place to rise for 1 hour.

3. Turn out dough onto a lightly floured work surface, using remaining whole-wheat flour as necessary. Gently punch down dough and divide into 6 equal pieces, forming into balls. Cover with plastic wrap coated with nonstick cooking spray, and let rest for 10 minutes.

4. Preheat the oven to 450°F. Place a large baking sheet in the preheating oven.

5. Flatten each dough ball on a lightly floured surface, using remaining whole-wheat flour as necessary. Roll out to 4- to 4½-inch circles about ⅛ inch thick. Cover with plastic wrap coated with nonstick cooking spray, and let rest for 10 minutes.

6. Quickly transfer dough to the hot baking sheet, and bake for 7 or 8 minutes or until puffed up and edges are browned. Cool on the baking sheet on a wire rack. To serve, cut into the edge of the pita pocket to open.

PINCH OF SAGE

You can create a warm environment for bread rising by turning the light on in your oven. Set your covered bread dough on the center rack, and keep the oven light on and the oven door closed during the rising time.

Whole-Wheat Sandwich Flats

This dense, whole-grain bun gives you a thin bread to close your sandwich while letting the flavors of your fillings shine.

Yield:	Prep time:	Rise time:	Cook time:	Serving size:
8 sandwich flats	25 minutes	1 hour, 20 minutes	6 minutes	1 sandwich flat
Each serving has:				
168.1 calories	2 mg sodium			

1 tsp. active dry yeast for whole grains

1 cup lukewarm water (100°F to 110°F)

1 tsp. granulated sugar

1 TB. extra-virgin olive oil

3 cups whole-wheat flour

1. In a medium bowl, dissolve yeast in lukewarm water. Stir in sugar and extra-virgin olive oil. Work in whole-wheat flour with a wooden spoon to incorporate as much as possible (about 2⅔ cups) to produce a cohesive dough ball.

2. Turn out dough onto a lightly floured work surface, using remaining whole-wheat flour as necessary. *Knead* for 8 to 10 minutes or until smooth and elastic. Work dough into a ball and transfer to a large bowl sprayed with nonstick cooking spray, turning dough over to coat. Cover with a clean dishcloth, and set in a warm place to rise for 1 hour.

3. Turn out dough onto a lightly floured work surface, using remaining whole-wheat flour as necessary. Gently punch down dough and divide into 8 equal pieces, forming into balls. Cover with plastic wrap coated with nonstick cooking spray, and let rest for 10 minutes.

4. Preheat the oven to 450°F. Place 2 large baking sheets in the preheating oven.

5. Flatten each dough ball on a lightly floured surface, using remaining whole-wheat flour as necessary. Roll out to 4-inch circles about ¼ inch thick. Cover with plastic wrap coated with nonstick cooking spray, and let rest for 10 minutes.

6. Quickly transfer dough to the hot baking sheets, and bake for 6 or 7 minutes or until slightly puffed and edges are browned. Cool slightly on the baking sheets on wire racks before serving. To serve, cut in half horizontally with a serrated knife.

DEFINITION

Knead bread dough on a lightly floured work surface with lightly floured hands by pushing into the dough ball with the heel of your hand, folding the dough back toward you, and rotating a quarter turn. Repeat this process for the time indicated by the recipe, lightly flouring the work surface and your hands as needed.

Basic Yeast Rolls

Soft and airy, these traditional dinner rolls make a tasty accompaniment to many dishes.

Yield:	Prep time:	Rise time:	Cook time:	Serving size:
14 rolls	30 minutes	2 hours	10 minutes	1 roll

Each serving has:		
126.9 calories	5.4 mg sodium	

1 (.25-oz.) pkg. active dry yeast	1½ TB. trans-fat-free vegetable shortening
1 cup lukewarm water (100°F to 110°F)	3 cups all-purpose flour
¼ cup granulated sugar	1 large egg, slightly beaten

1. In a large bowl, dissolve yeast in lukewarm water. Stir in sugar and vegetable shortening. Alternately add flour and egg with a wooden spoon until dough forms and starts to clean the side of the bowl.

2. Cover dough with a clean dishcloth. Set in a warm place, and let rise for 30 minutes. Punch down dough. Cover with plastic wrap, and chill. Punch down dough 2 or 3 times every 30 to 60 minutes.

3. When ready to bake, turn out dough onto a lightly floured work surface, incorporating just enough flour to keep it from being too tacky. Roll out dough to about a ½-inch thickness. Cut out rolls with a 2½-inch cutter, and place on large nonstick baking sheets at least 1 inch apart. Cover with clean dishcloths, and let rest for 10 minutes.

4. Meanwhile, preheat the oven to 350°F.

5. Bake rolls for 10 or 11 minutes or until lightly browned.

 PINCH OF SAGE

You can hold this dough in the refrigerator for several hours until you're ready to bake the rolls. Time when you'll punch down the chilled dough to meet your intended baking time.

Banana Chocolate-Chip Muffins

Loaded with chocolate chips, these hearty muffins boast undertones of banana flavor.

Yield:	Prep time:	Cook time:	Serving size:
12 muffins	15 minutes	25 minutes	1 muffin

Each serving has:			
316.4 calories	6 mg sodium		

1 cup all-purpose flour	½ cup honey
1 cup whole-wheat flour	⅓ cup canola oil
1 cup ground flaxseed	1 large egg, beaten
1 TB. sodium-free baking powder	1 tsp. vanilla extract
1 cup mashed ripe bananas (about 3 medium)	1 cup miniature semisweet chocolate chips

1. Preheat the oven to 350°F. Spray a 12-cup muffin pan with nonstick cooking spray.

2. In a large bowl, combine all-purpose flour, whole-wheat flour, ground flaxseed, and sodium-free baking powder. Stir to mix.

3. In a medium bowl, combine mashed bananas and honey, and stir until blended. Add canola oil, egg, and vanilla extract, and stir to blend.

4. Add chocolate chips to flour mixture, and stir to coat. Add banana mixture, and stir just until moistened.

5. Working quickly, spoon batter into the prepared muffin cups, filling each ⅞ full. Bake for 25 minutes or until a cake tester inserted into the center of muffin comes out clean.

6. Cool in the pan on a wire rack for 10 minutes. Remove muffins, and cool completely on the wire rack. Store any leftovers in an airtight container in the refrigerator for 4 or 5 days.

SALT PITFALL

When using sodium-free baking powder, keep the dry ingredients separated from the wet ingredients for as long as possible. Once you add the liquid ingredient(s) to the sodium-free baking powder, you need to work quickly to ensure the baked goods will rise as intended.

Old Welsh Speckled Bread

Known as *bara brith* in Wales, this fruit-studded loaf is reminiscent of fruit cake, but lighter as a quick bread.

Yield:	Prep time:	Soak time:	Cook time:	Serving size:
16 servings	12 minutes	6 to 8 hours	90 minutes	1 (½-inch-thick) slice

Each serving has:	
152.2 calories	6.2 mg sodium

3 green tea bags

1 cup boiling water

¾ cup honey

1½ cups dried mixed fruit (dates, dried cranberries, raisins, golden raisins)

1¾ cups all-purpose flour

1½ tsp. sodium-free baking powder

¼ tsp. sodium-free baking soda

1 tsp. ground cinnamon

1 tsp. pumpkin pie spice mix

1 large egg, at room temperature

1. In a medium bowl, brew tea bags in boiling water for 5 minutes. Remove tea bags, pressing out water into the bowl.

2. Stir in honey until dissolved. Stir in dried mixed fruit, cover loosely, and soak for 6 to 8 hours or overnight.

3. Preheat the oven to 325°F. Line the bottom of a 9×5×2 loaf pan with parchment paper, and coat the pan with nonstick cooking spray.

4. In a large bowl, stir together all-purpose flour, sodium-free baking powder, sodium-free baking soda, cinnamon, and pumpkin pie spice mix.

5. In a small bowl, lightly beat egg. Stir egg and fruit mixture into flour mixture just until moistened. Immediately pour into the prepared pan. Bake for 90 to 100 minutes or until a cake tester comes out clean when inserted in the center. Cool on a wire rack for 10 minutes.

6. Turn out of loaf pan, and continue cooling on a wire rack. Slice with a serrated knife to serve.

PINCH OF SAGE

Bring any eggs called for in baking to room temperature before adding to the batter. Room-temperature eggs blend better than do refrigerator-cold eggs.

Classic Cornmeal Biscuits

Round out your meal with a mild taste of cornmeal in a hearty biscuit.

Yield:	Prep time:	Cook time:	Serving size:
1 dozen	15 minutes	11 minutes	1 biscuit
Each serving has:			
130.9 calories	7.8 mg sodium		

1½ cups all-purpose flour

½ cup yellow cornmeal

2 tsp. sodium-free baking powder

⅓ cup trans-fat-free vegetable shortening

⅔ cup fat-free milk

1. Preheat the oven to 450°F. Spray a baking sheet with nonstick cooking spray.

2. In a large bowl, stir together flour, cornmeal, and baking powder. Using a pastry blender, 2 knives, or your fingertips, cut in vegetable shortening until coarse crumbs form. Stir in milk with a fork until moistened and dough cleans the side of the bowl.

3. Lightly sprinkle additional cornmeal onto a work surface, and pat dough to ½-inch thickness. Cut biscuits with a 2-inch cutter, and place on the prepared baking sheet. Bake for 11 to 14 minutes or until lightly browned and raised.

PINCH OF SAGE

If you don't have a 2-inch biscuit cutter or a round cookie cutter, in a pinch, you can use the top of a glass.

Tangy Glazed Lemon Bread

Sink your teeth into this moist quick bread with a sweet-tart syrupy topping.

Yield:	Prep time:	Cook time:	Serving size:
12 servings	20 minutes	50 minutes	1 slice
Each serving has:			
226 calories	16.5 mg sodium		

6 TB. unsalted butter, melted	$\frac{1}{2}$ cup unsalted chopped walnuts
1 cup granulated sugar	1 cup all-purpose flour
2 large eggs, at room temperature	$\frac{1}{2}$ cup whole-wheat flour
$\frac{1}{2}$ cup fat-free milk	2 TB. fresh lemon juice
1 tsp. sodium-free baking powder	2 TB. confectioners' sugar
1 TB. grated lemon zest	

1. Preheat the oven to 350°F. Grease a 9×5×3-inch nonstick loaf pan with nonstick cooking spray with flour.

2. In a large mixing bowl, blend butter and sugar. Add eggs, and beat until thoroughly blended. Add milk, baking powder, lemon zest, and walnuts, and mix well.

3. Add all-purpose flour and whole-wheat flour, mixing just until moistened.

4. Turn batter into the prepared pan, and spread evenly into the corners. Bake for 50 to 55 minutes or until a cake tester inserted in the center comes out clean.

5. Meanwhile, in a small bowl, stir together lemon juice and confectioners' sugar.

6. Remove the loaf pan to a wire rack. With the tines of a large fork, poke holes all over the top of loaf. Stir lemon juice mixture, and pour over top of loaf. Cool in the pan for 15 minutes. Remove loaf from the pan, and cool completely on a wire rack.

PINCH OF SAGE

A medium lemon yields about 1 tablespoon zest and 2 tablespoons juice, perfect for this recipe. If you need both the zest and the juice from a lemon, grate the zest before squeezing the juice.

Sweet Wheat Buns

You'll love these lightly wheaty-tasting morsels with extra sweetness baked in a crisped crust.

Yield:	Prep time:	Rise time:	Cook time:	Serving size:
1½ dozen	25 minutes	1 hour	15 minutes	1 bun

Each serving has:				
181.9 calories	21.7 mg sodium			

3 cups unbleached all-purpose flour	½ cup unsalted butter
1 cup whole-wheat flour	4 large eggs, at room temperature
1 (.25-oz.) pkg. active dry yeast	2 tsp. lemon extract
1 cup fat-free milk	5 TB. granulated sugar

1. In a large bowl, stir together all-purpose flour and whole-wheat flour. Add yeast, and stir to combine. Make a well in center of dry ingredients.

2. In a small saucepan over medium heat, heat milk and butter to 120°F, stirring to melt butter.

3. Add eggs to well in dry ingredients. Pour in milk mixture, and add lemon extract. Beat with a wooden spoon until well combined and elastic. Cover bowl with a clean dishcloth, and set in a warm place to rise for 1 hour.

4. Preheat the oven to 400°F. Spray 2 large baking sheets with nonstick cooking spray.

5. Turn out dough onto a lightly floured work surface, and using your fingers, gently and gradually work in sugar. Pinch off dough in pieces about the size of hockey pucks, and place on the prepared baking sheets. Cover with clean dishcloths, and let rest for 10 minutes.

6. Bake buns for 15 to 20 minutes or until browned and done.

PINCH OF SAGE

For even baking, rotate your baking pans from front to back and from the top rack to the bottom rack halfway through the baking time.

Easy Spoon Bread

Serve up this soft, custardy cornbread with a spoon.

Yield:	Prep time:	Cook time:	Serving size:
6 servings	20 minutes	45 minutes	1 wedge

Each serving has:		
170.2 calories	53.4 mg sodium	

2 cups water	4 large eggs
1 cup yellow cornmeal	$\frac{1}{2}$ cup fat-free milk
2 TB. unsalted butter	

1. Preheat the oven to 400°F. Grease an 8-inch-round casserole dish with nonstick cooking spray with flour.

2. In a medium saucepan over high heat, bring water to a boil. Slowly stir in cornmeal, reduce heat to low, and cook, stirring, for 5 minutes. Remove from heat and let stand for 5 to 10 minutes to cool slightly.

3. Add butter to the saucepan.

4. In a small bowl, beat eggs with milk. Add to the saucepan, and stir cornmeal mixture until blended. Turn into the prepared dish.

5. Bake for 40 to 45 minutes or until top is browned and bread is done. Serve hot, cutting into wedges.

PINCH OF SAGE

You may want to serve this custard-style bread with the gravy or meat juices from your meal. It's also good served with butter or syrup.

Apple Raisin Bread

This cinnamon-spiced, airy quick bread packs apple flavor in every plumped raisin.

Yield:	Prep time:	Cook time:	Serving size:
12 servings	20 minutes	1 hour	1 slice
Each serving has:			
270.1 calories	74.2 mg sodium		

¾ cup dark raisins

¼ cup natural apple juice

1½ cups all-purpose flour

1 cup quick oats

¾ cup light brown sugar, firmly packed

1½ tsp. sodium-free baking powder

½ tsp. sodium-free baking soda

1½ tsp. ground cinnamon

1¼ cups unsweetened applesauce

⅓ cup extra-light olive oil

2 large eggs, beaten

¼ cup fat-free milk

1. Preheat the oven to 350°F. Grease the bottom of an 8½×4½-inch nonstick loaf pan with nonstick cooking spray with flour.

2. In a small bowl, soak raisins in apple juice. Set aside.

3. In a large bowl, stir together flour, oats, light brown sugar, baking powder, baking soda, and cinnamon. Add applesauce, extra-light olive oil, eggs, and milk, and stir just until dry ingredients are moistened. Stir in raisin mixture.

4. Pour batter into the prepared pan. Bake for 60 to 65 minutes or until top is browned and a cake tester inserted in the center comes out clean. Remove to a wire rack to cool for 10 minutes. Remove loaf from the pan, and cool completely on a wire rack.

PINCH OF SAGE

You'll find nonstick cooking spray with flour in your grocer's baking aisle next to the regular nonstick cooking spray. It's great for easy, one-step coating. If you can't find nonstick cooking spray with flour, you can spray the pan with regular nonstick cooking spray and lightly dust the pan with flour, shaking out any excess flour.

Sweet Strawberry Bread

This pink-tinged, light quick bread is filled with strawberry goodness.

Yield:	Prep time:	Cook time:	Serving size:
12 servings	30 minutes	55 minutes	1 slice

Each serving has:			
231.1 calories	116.7 mg sodium		

1 (16-oz.) pkg. unsweetened frozen strawberries, thawed	2 large eggs, separated
½ cup unsalted butter, softened	2 cups all-purpose flour
1 cup granulated sugar	1 tsp. sodium-free baking powder
½ tsp. pure almond extract	1 tsp. sodium-free baking soda

1. Preheat the oven to 350°F. Grease a 9×5×3-inch nonstick loaf pan with nonstick cooking spray with flour.

2. Drain strawberries well, reserving ¼ cup juice. Chop strawberries and set aside.

3. In a large bowl, and using an electric mixer on medium speed, mix butter, sugar, and almond extract for 2 or 3 minutes or until well blended. Add egg yolks, and beat until well blended. On low speed, mix in flour, baking powder, and baking soda until fine crumbs form.

4. Stir in reserved strawberry juice by hand until evenly distributed. Fold in strawberries until blended.

5. In a small bowl, and using an electric mixer on medium speed, beat egg whites until frothy. Increase speed to high, and beat until stiff peaks form. Fold egg whites into strawberry mixture until blended.

6. Turn batter into the prepared pan, pushing into the corners. *Tamp* pan lightly. Bake for 55 to 60 minutes or until a cake tester inserted in the center comes out clean. Cool in the pan for 15 minutes on a wire rack. Remove from pan, and cool completely on wire rack.

DEFINITION

Tamp means to tap the baking pan on the counter a few times to release any air bubbles from the batter.

The Salad Bar

In This Chapter

- Reaping the rewards of nutritious salads
- Filling your diet with veggies and fruits
- Topping with low-sodium dressings
- Easy-to-prepare side salads

Many meals begin with a salad, even if it's as simple as a small tossed green salad with a couple vegetables. This custom is well founded, as easily prepared salads supply plenty of vitamins, minerals, antioxidants, and fiber.

What makes an ordinary salad extraordinary is a great-tasting dressing. With a salad dressing as equally healthful as the salad it enhances, you can confidently relish in its goodness. Many salad dressings are high in sodium, so keep an eye on that. The recipes that follow keep your sodium intake in check while allowing you an ample assortment of side salads.

Easy to prepare, packed with nutrients, readily made low in sodium—no wonder salads open meals so often.

Greens and Beans

A great green salad or bean salad allows a healthful foundation to a satisfying meal. And beginning your meal with a filling salad can keep you from overindulging in less-nutritious offerings.

The green salads shared in this chapter call for spring mix greens, baby spinach, butter lettuce, and radicchio. But you don't have to stick to these greens. You can substitute a wide variety of greens, from what you have in the crisper that needs to be used up, to specially selected lettuces. Give Bibb lettuce, romaine, Belgian endive, peppery arugula, escarole, red leaf lettuce, or even standard iceberg lettuce a try.

The same goes for bean salads. You can substitute any number of no-salt-added canned beans or cooked dried beans. Maybe you love limas, Great Northern beans, pinto beans, adzuki beans, navy beans, or others. Mix them up to keep your taste buds tantalized.

PINCH OF SAGE

Dress green salads just before serving to prevent the salad greens from wilting. If you have to hold a salad, keep the dressing separate until serving time.

Pasta Possibilities

Pasta salads are comforting foods, often dressed in rich, creamy salad dressings. As long as you keep the portion size in check, you can easily indulge in their homey feeling.

Any pasta salad can be made with a variety of shapes. If you have a different pasta shape in your pantry or simply prefer to use something other than the shape called for, you can—just keep a few guidelines in mind.

A substitute should be the same size as the shape called for. Popular small cuts are orzo, acini de pepe, and small shells. Favorite medium shapes are rotini, bow ties (also known as farfalle), elbow macaroni, and wagon wheels. Various large pastas such as manicotti and jumbo shells can be stuffed with salad mixtures. Pasta strands vary in thickness or width, ranging from very dainty angel hair to spaghetti, as well as from linguini to fettuccini.

Heavy or chunky salads and sauces need substantial carriers. Try radiatore, penne, rigatoni, and fusilli. Lighter salads and thinner sauces complement smooth, delicate pasta varieties, such as ditalini and vermicelli.

Whole-wheat pastas continue to grow in popularity and are becoming available in a wider array of shapes. Choose whole-wheat varieties to increase your whole-grain consumption.

With a low-sodium dressing to coat and the addition of healthful fruits and veggies, pasta salads can be an appetizing way to add a nutritious side dish to any meal.

Fantastic Fruit

If you're not partial to eating raw fruit out of hand, a prepared fruit salad is a tasty way to reach your recommended 2 cups fruit a day for a 2,000-calorie diet. You can serve a fruit salad as an appetizing first course or a scrumptious side dish. Many fruit salads make mouthwatering desserts as well for a nutritious, naturally sweet ending to an everyday meal.

Fruit salads are also perfect for any number of gatherings. Luncheon, shower, and reunion guests happily welcome the fresh taste. The good news for you is that the fruitastic recipes in this chapter are easy to prepare.

Pearly Fruit Salad

Juicy bites of apples, oranges, and grapes team up with the tang of yogurt in this pasta salad.

Yield:	Prep time:	Cook time:	Chill time:	Serving size:
2 cups	5 minutes	10 minutes	4 hours	¹⁄₂ cup

Each serving has:	
58.1 calories	5.5 mg sodium

¹⁄₃ cup *acini de pepe* pasta

2 TB. fat-free plain yogurt

¹⁄₂ medium Gala or other apple, skin on, cored, and finely chopped

¹⁄₃ cup drained mandarin orange sections

10 seedless green grapes, halved

1. In a small saucepan, cook pasta according to the package directions (omit salt). Rinse under cold water, and drain thoroughly.

2. In a small bowl, stir yogurt into apple pieces to coat. Stir in mandarin orange sections and grapes. Stir pasta (about 1 cup cooked) into fruit mixture.

3. Chill for at least 4 hours before serving.

DEFINITION

Italian for "peppercorns," **acini de pepe** is a small pasta, sometimes grouped with pastinas (see note in Chapter 7). The tiny, beadlike pasta is commonly used in soups and cold salads.

Melon Berry Cups

Summer-fresh fruits enjoy a citrusy splash of lime.

Yield:	Prep time:	Serving size:
7 cups	10 minutes	½ cup
Each serving has:		
50.1 calories	8.1 mg sodium	

2 TB. fresh lime juice	6 cups bite-size honeydew chunks
¼ cup honey	1 cup fresh blueberries

1. In a large bowl, stir together lime juice and honey until well blended. Stir in honey-dew until well coated. Gently stir in blueberries until thoroughly combined.

2. Serve immediately or refrigerate until serving time, serving in individual serving cups as desired.

Salternative: If you're not using this salad as a carry-in dish, decrease the recipe as needed.

SALT PITFALL

Don't feed honey to children younger than 1 year old. The digestive systems of infants may be too immature to digest possibly present bacterial spores, which can make the babies sick.

Tropical White Tie Salad

An assortment of sweet fruits are coated with a tart, fruit-flavored yogurt in this pasta salad.

Yield:	Prep time:	Cook time:	Chill time:	Serving size:
8 cups	20 minutes	10 minutes	4 hours	⅔ cup

Each serving has:	
113.3 calories	10.9 mg sodium

2 cups bow-tie pasta

2 medium kiwifruit, peeled, halved, and sliced

2 cups chopped fresh pineapple

1 cup seedless red or green grapes

2 medium Braeburn apples, skin on, cored, and chopped

1 (6-oz.) container fat-free, sugar-free strawberry-banana yogurt

¼ cup unsweetened orange juice

1. Cook pasta according to the package directions (omit salt). Rinse under cold water, and drain thoroughly.

2. In a large bowl, combine kiwifruit, pineapple, grapes, and apples.

3. In a small bowl, stir together yogurt and orange juice until blended. Pour over fruit mixture, and stir to coat. Add pasta, and stir until evenly coated.

4. Cover and chill for at least 4 hours before serving. Stir again before serving.

PINCH OF SAGE

If you find this salad too tart, stir a little honey into the yogurt mixture.

Tangy Lemon Waldorf Salad

The traditional apple, walnut, and raisin combination is dressed with a lemon-flavored yogurt.

Yield:	Prep time:	Chill time:	Serving size:
5 cups	20 minutes	1 hour	½ cup

Each serving has:	
60 calories	11.8 mg sodium

3 small McIntosh apples, skin on, cored, and finely chopped

1 (6-oz.) container fat-free, sugar-free lemon yogurt

1 small rib celery, diced

¼ cup dark raisins

¼ cup chopped unsalted walnuts

1. In a medium bowl, stir apples into yogurt. Stir in celery, raisins, and walnuts until evenly coated.

2. Chill for at least 1 hour before serving. Stir again before serving on plates lined with lettuce leaves, if desired.

PINCH OF SAGE

It's best to prepare this salad the same day as you serve it. The apples will weep and discolor if held for a day or two.

Zesty Vinaigrette Coleslaw

Wilted cabbage is spiced up with a blush of heat.

Yield:	Prep time:	Chill time:	Serving size:
3 cups	5 minutes	2 hours	½ cup
Each serving has:			
109.1 calories	12.2 mg sodium		

3 cups coarsely shredded green
    cabbage

½ cup shredded carrots

½ cup thinly sliced and halved red
    onions

3 TB. cider vinegar

3 TB. extra-virgin olive oil

2 TB. honey

¼ tsp. cayenne

¼ tsp. dry mustard

¼ tsp. garlic powder

¼ tsp. freshly ground black pepper

1. In a large bowl, combine cabbage, carrots, and red onions.

2. In a small bowl, combine cider vinegar, extra-virgin olive oil, honey, cayenne, dry mustard, garlic powder, and pepper. Whisk until well blended.

3. Pour vinegar mixture over cabbage mixture, and stir to coat evenly. Cover and chill for at least 2 hours before serving. Stir again before serving.

PINCH OF SAGE

Cayenne gives this salad a blush and your body a small dose of minerals, vitamins, and phytonutrients that may promote your health.

Busy-Day Ambrosia

Honey-sweetened fruits are enlivened with a tropical touch of coconut.

Yield:	Prep time:	Serving size:
3 cups	10 minutes	½ cup
Each serving has:		
134.6 calories	13.5 mg sodium	

2 (11-oz.) cans mandarin orange sections, drained (½ cup liquid reserved)

¼ cup honey

2 TB. fresh lemon juice

2 medium bananas, peeled and sliced

¼ cup sweetened flaked coconut

1. In a small bowl, combine reserved mandarin orange liquid, honey, and lemon juice. Stir until blended.

2. In a medium bowl, combine mandarin orange sections and bananas. Pour honey mixture over top, and stir. Sprinkle coconut over top.

3. Serve immediately, or chill briefly until serving time.

Crunchy Cucumber Salad

Crisp cucumbers and nutty almond bits pair with a tangy chive-enhanced yogurt dressing.

Yield:	Prep time:	Serving size:
2 cups	15 minutes	½ cup
Each serving has:		
83.3 calories	16.9 mg sodium	

½ cup fat-free plain yogurt

¼ cup unsalted chopped almonds

2 TB. chopped fresh chives or 2 tsp. dried

½ tsp. fresh lemon juice

1½ medium cucumbers, peeled and very thinly sliced

1. In a medium bowl, combine yogurt, almonds, chives, and lemon juice. Stir until well blended.

2. Add cucumbers to yogurt mixture, and gently stir until evenly coated. Serve immediately, or cover and chill until serving time.

Salternative: Season the cucumbers with Salt-Shaker Substitute (recipe in Chapter 14) or another salt-free salt substitute seasoning blend if you like.

Homey Macaroni Salad

This classic pasta-and-egg salad provides the crunch of veggies in a yogurt-based sauce with a hint of tang.

Yield:	Prep time:	Chill time:	Serving size:
9 cups	10 minutes	4 hours	½ cup
Each serving has:			
146.6 calories	18.7 mg sodium		

4 cups elbow macaroni pasta (8 cups cooked)

2 large hard-boiled eggs, finely chopped

½ medium green bell pepper, ribs and seeds removed, and finely diced

¼ cup minced yellow onions

1¾ cups Classic Potato Salad Dressing (recipe in Chapter 6)

¼ tsp. celery seed

¼ tsp. freshly ground black pepper

1. Cook pasta according to the package directions (omit salt). Rinse under cold water, and drain thoroughly.

2. In a large bowl, combine pasta, hard-boiled eggs, green bell pepper, and onions. Stir in Classic Potato Salad Dressing, celery seed, and pepper. Mix well.

3. Cover and chill for at least 4 hours or until thoroughly chilled before serving.

Salternative: This salad makes a great picnic dish for a crowd, but you can halve the recipe easily for a smaller yield.

PINCH OF SAGE

Hard-boiling is a great way to prepare older eggs. (Eggs can be used for up to 3 to 5 weeks after the sell-by date.) Don't choose new eggs for hard-boiling; peeling them is nearly impossible.

Layered Sweet Banana Salad

Fruity bananas and crunchy peanuts are layered with a sweet brown sugar sauce.

Yield:	Prep time:	Cook time:	Serving size:
4 cups	10 minutes	8 minutes	½ cup

Each serving has:		
229.6 calories	19 mg sodium	

1 cup firmly packed light brown sugar

1 large egg, beaten

1½ TB. white vinegar

3½ TB. water

1 TB. unsalted butter

5 medium bananas, peeled and sliced

⅓ cup chopped unsalted peanuts

1. In a medium saucepan over high heat, combine light brown sugar, egg, white vinegar, and water. Bring to a boil, stirring constantly. Reduce heat to medium, and cook, stirring, for 5 to 7 minutes or until thickened. Remove from heat, and stir in butter.

2. In a serving dish, alternately layer bananas, light brown sugar mixture, and peanuts as your serving dish allows. Serve warm or at room temperature.

SALT PITFALL

Stir steadily while bringing the brown sugar mixture to a boil or you'll risk cooking the egg instead of blending it into the mixture.

Creamy Avocado and Pink Grapefruit Toss

Tart grapefruit stands out against the smooth richness of avocados.

Yield:	Prep time:	Serving size:
6 cups	10 minutes	1½ cups

Each serving has:		
145.5 calories	20.1 mg sodium	

4 cups mixed butter lettuce and radicchio salad greens

1 medium pink grapefruit, peeled and sectioned

1 medium ripe avocado, peeled, pitted, and sliced

½ cup Creamy Avocado Dressing (recipe in Chapter 6)

1. Line each of 4 plates with 1 cup salad greens. Scatter ¼ grapefruit sections and ¼ avocado slices on top.

2. Serve each salad with 2 tablespoons Creamy Avocado Dressing, and serve immediately.

PINCH OF SAGE

To prevent the avocado slices from discoloring, rub them all over with a little fresh lemon juice.

Crunchy Apple Coleslaw

This creamy slaw features the surprise crunch of crisp apples and almonds.

Yield:	Prep time:	Chill time:	Serving size:
3½ cups	10 minutes	1 hour	½ cup
Each serving has:			
65.7 calories	25.8 mg sodium		

½ cup fat-free sugar-free vanilla
  yogurt

½ cup fat-free sour cream

1 medium Golden Delicious apple,
  unpeeled, cored, and diced

2 cups shredded red cabbage

¼ cup unsalted slivered almonds

1. In a medium bowl, blend together yogurt and sour cream. Stir in apple to coat. Stir in red cabbage and almonds until evenly coated.

2. Cover and chill for at least 1 hour before serving. Stir again before serving.

Herbed Baby Greens Side Salad

Simple spring greens are topped with red onion rings and crisp seasoned croutons.

Yield:	Prep time:	Serving size:
1 serving	2 minutes	1 salad
Each serving has:		
70 calories	30.5 mg sodium	

1 cup torn mixed baby salad
  greens, lightly packed

1 TB. coarsely chopped fresh basil

1 TB. coarsely chopped fresh
  parsley

1 thin slice red onion, separated
  into rings

¼ cup Garlic-Pepper Croutons
  (recipe in Chapter 6)

1. In an individual serving bowl, combine mixed baby salad greens, basil, and parsley. Toss well.

2. Arrange red onion rings and Garlic-Pepper Croutons on top. Serve with 1 tablespoon of your favorite low-sodium salad dressing, if desired.

PINCH OF SAGE

To add the least amount of salad dressing to a salad, toss your greens (and other ingredients) with a little salad dressing to coat the leaves evenly, distributing the flavor and reducing the puddling.

Frosty Apricot Salad

This frozen treat is smooth and fruity with a crunch of peanut pieces.

Yield:	Prep time:	Freeze time:	Serving size:
9 servings	15 minutes	4 hours	2½×2½-inch square
Each serving has:			
97.7 calories	33.4 mg sodium		

3 (6-oz.) containers fat-free, sugar-free orange crème yogurt	1 lb. fresh apricots, skin on, halved and pitted
1 TB. grated orange zest	½ cup chopped unsalted peanuts

1. In a medium bowl, stir together yogurt and orange zest until combined.

2. Cut each apricot half into 4 slices. Stir apricot slices and peanuts into yogurt mixture. Turn into an 8×8×2-inch casserole dish that's been sprayed with nonstick cooking spray.

3. Freeze for 4 hours or until firm. Cut into squares to serve, arranging on lettuce-lined salad plates, as desired.

PINCH OF SAGE

For easier cutting, remove this frozen salad from the freezer about 10 minutes before serving time.

Grape and Walnut Spinach Salad

Sweet fruit and crunchy nuts mingle in this fresh spinach salad tossed with a sweet and creamy dressing.

Yield:	Prep time:	Serving size:
4 cups	10 minutes	½ cup
Each serving has:		
122.1 calories	40.1 mg sodium	

1 (6-oz.) pkg. baby spinach (about 3 cups)	1 cup unsalted walnut halves and pieces
1½ cups halved seedless green grapes	6 TB. Creamy Herb Dressing (recipe in Chapter 6)

1. In a large salad bowl, combine spinach, grapes, and walnuts.

2. Drizzle Creamy Herb Dressing over salad, and toss until evenly coated.

Crimson-Jeweled Baby Spinach Salad

Sweet cranberries and mandarin oranges perk up this fresh spinach salad with a crunch of walnuts.

Yield:	Prep time:	Serving size:
6 cups	30 minutes	1 cup
Each serving has:		
208.7 calories	50.4 mg sodium	

2 TB. white wine vinegar	¼ tsp. ground nutmeg
3 TB. extra-virgin olive oil	½ cup dried cranberries
2 (11-oz.) cans mandarin orange sections, drained (reserve 3 TB. liquid)	1 (6-oz.) pkg. baby spinach leaves (about 3 cups)
	½ cup unsalted walnut pieces

1. In a large salad bowl, combine white wine vinegar, extra-virgin olive oil, reserved mandarin orange liquid, and nutmeg. Whisk until blended.

2. Stir in dried cranberries, and toss to coat. Let stand for at least 20 minutes.

3. Stir in mandarin oranges. Add spinach, and toss to coat completely. Toss in walnut pieces. Serve immediately, or hold in refrigerator until serving time.

SALT PITFALL

Spinach, as well as other dark leafy greens such as kale and turnip greens, is a bit higher in sodium than many other vegetables. However, these greens are packed with nutrients, so include them, as you're able, in a healthful diet and enjoy their power-packed nutritional punch. Still other dark leafy greens, such as beet greens and chicory greens, are much higher in sodium. Ask your doctor or nutritionist if these greens can be a part of your sodium-restricted diet.

Cowboy Rice and Black Bean Salad

With a hint of jalapeño heat, this rice-based salad serves up the big Texas taste of beans with cilantro and lime.

Yield:	Prep time:	Chill time:	Serving size:
6⅔ cups	20 minutes	8 hours	⅔ cup
Each serving has:			
97.3 calories	90.7 mg sodium		

2 cups cooked long-grain brown rice

1 (15-oz.) can no-salt-added black beans, rinsed and drained

2 cups frozen whole-kernel corn

1 medium red bell pepper, ribs and seeds removed, and chopped

1 small yellow onion, diced

1 medium fresh jalapeño pepper, ribs and seeds removed, and minced

¼ cup cider vinegar

1½ TB. fresh lime juice

¼ cup chopped fresh cilantro

1 tsp. Firehouse Chili Powder (recipe in Chapter 14) or other salt-free chili powder

1. In a large bowl, combine rice, black beans, corn, red bell pepper, onion, jalapeño pepper, cider vinegar, lime juice, cilantro, and Firehouse Chili Powder. Stir to mix thoroughly.

2. Cover and chill overnight. Stir again before serving.

PINCH OF SAGE

Store limes in the refrigerator, but return them to room temperature before juicing to extract more juice. If you're rushed, pop the lime into the microwave for 3 to 10 seconds or just until the chill is taken off.

Basic Three-Bean Salad

A mildly spicy vinaigrette marinates this classic bean medley.

Yield:	Prep time:	Chill time:	Serving size:
5 cups	20 minutes	2 hours	½ cup
Each serving has:			
139.2 calories	98.1 mg sodium		

½ cup cider vinegar

¼ cup extra-virgin olive oil

1 TB. honey

½ tsp. dry mustard

¼ tsp. garlic powder

¼ tsp. onion powder

¼ tsp. ground black pepper

¼ tsp. cayenne

1 (15-oz.) can no-salt-added green beans, drained and rinsed

1 (15-oz.) can no-salt-added cannellini beans, drained and rinsed

1 (15-oz.) can low-sodium chickpeas, drained and rinsed

4 medium green onions, trimmed and thinly sliced

1 rib celery, finely diced

1. In a large bowl, combine cider vinegar, extra-virgin olive oil, honey, dry mustard, garlic powder, onion powder, pepper, and cayenne. Whisk until well blended.

2. Add green beans, cannellini beans, chickpeas, green onions, and celery, and gently stir to coat.

3. Cover and chill for at least 2 hours before serving. Stir again before serving.

PINCH OF SAGE

You can use any three-bean combination you prefer for this salad—just choose the no-salt-added or low-sodium varieties.

Spring Mix with Sun-Dried Tomatoes and Fresh Mozzarella

The sharp bite of sun-dried tomatoes balances the smooth mozzarella slices drizzled with a sweet balsamic vinaigrette.

Yield:	Prep time:	Serving size:
2⅔ cups	10 minutes	⅔ cup

Each serving has:		
193.5 calories	292.9 mg sodium	

2 cups spring mix greens	4 oz. fresh mozzarella cheese, sliced
8 dry-packed sun-dried tomatoes, rehydrated	¼ cup Balsamic Vinaigrette (recipe in Chapter 6)

1. On each of 4 salad plates, arrange ½ cup greens, 2 sun-dried tomatoes, and 1 ounce mozzarella cheese.

2. Drizzle 1 tablespoon Balsamic Vinaigrette over each salad.

PINCH OF SAGE

To rehydrate the sun-dried tomatoes, cover them with boiling hot water. Let stand for 5 minutes or until plumped, and drain.

À la Carte Items

In This Chapter

- Simple yet spectacular side dishes
- Salt-free vegetable sides
- Perfect pasta sides
- Great grain and rice sides

After deciding on what to cook for dinner, do you know what you'll serve beyond the entrée? Are you in such a rut that when you tell your family you're having fish, they expect to see rice pilaf, green beans, and carrots on the table as well? If you usually give little thought to side dishes, let your need for low-sodium foods be the impetus to planning a full, harmonized meal.

Side dishes can be satisfying and delicious. More importantly, all your side dishes can fit into your sodium-restricted diet. Veggies, noodles, and grains are good vehicles for spices, herbs, and other flavorings. You may enjoy some of these side dishes so much that you'll decide on dinner in relation to what entrée complements them best! Or just make a meal of several sides—who needs an entrée?

Veggie Venue

If you've grown accustomed to steaming a couple vegetables and shaking on salt and pepper, you'll be relieved to learn that you can prepare tasty veggies just as easily without adding salt. The simple addition of lemon juice, herbs, or unsalted nuts can easily liven up your veggies. You can choose more involved sides as well when you have the time or occasion.

Because vegetables are so easy to prepare, make several—of various colors—to complete each meal. This is an easy way to reach the 2½ cups vegetables recommended for a 2,000-calorie daily diet.

> **PINCH OF SAGE**
>
> If you're a die-hard salt-and-pepper vegetable seasoner, veggies are a great way to try out the various tastes of salt-free salt-substitute seasoning blends, including our Salt-Shaker Substitute (recipe in Chapter 14).

Noodles and Grains

Noodles and pastas are comfort foods that make a homemade meal feel homey. Of course, remember to prepare all your noodles and pastas without the optional salt called for in the package directions. You won't lose a bit of flavor either, as noodles are perfect blank canvases for seasonings.

Serving side dishes made with grains is a tasty way to add more whole grains to your diet. Once again, always cook any grain without the optional salt (or optional fat) suggested on the package.

You're probably familiar with rice, but other grains may be more foreign to you. Check out millet and buckwheat groats, or kasha (roasted buckwheat groats; find these in your grocer's grain and dried bean section). These, along with other grains you may find such as quinoa, barley, and bulgur, offer variety and great taste for your family.

Oven-Crisped Fries

Golden-brown and lightly seasoned, these natural potato sticks save on sodium and fat.

Yield:	Prep time:	Cook time:	Serving size:
1⅓ cups	5 minutes	20 minutes	⅔ cup

Each serving has:		
101.7 calories	0.2 mg sodium	

2 medium all-purpose potatoes	⅛ tsp. garlic powder
Nonstick cooking spray	Pinch ground white pepper
¼ tsp. onion powder	

1. Place the oven rack in the highest position. Preheat the oven to 400°F. Generously spray a nonstick baking sheet with nonstick cooking spray.

2. Cut potatoes into ¼-inch matchsticks. Arrange in a single layer on the prepared sheet. Spray with nonstick cooking spray to coat. Bake for 10 minutes. Turn potatoes, and bake for 10 minutes more or until crisp.

3. In a small dish, combine onion powder, garlic powder, and white pepper. Stir to combine. Sprinkle over fries, tossing to coat. Serve with Kitchen Ketchup (recipe in Chapter 12) or no-salt-added ketchup, if desired.

Salternative: Some people like to leave the skin on their potatoes when making fries. However, if you prefer skinless, feel free to peel the potatoes.

Classic Spaghetti with Garlic and Olive Oil

Garlic-infused olive oil quickly and simply coats spaghetti with great taste.

Yield:	Prep time:	Cook time:	Serving size:
2 cups	5 minutes	10 minutes	1/2 cup

Each serving has:		
143.5 calories	0.8 mg sodium	

4 oz. thin spaghetti or regular spaghetti

1 large clove garlic

1½ TB. extra-virgin olive oil

Pinch freshly ground black pepper

Snipped fresh parsley (optional)

1. Cook spaghetti according to the package directions (omit salt). Drain, reserving 1 or 2 tablespoons cooking water. Return spaghetti to the cooking pot.

2. Meanwhile, press garlic through a garlic press into a small skillet. Pour in extra-virgin olive oil, and heat over medium-low heat for 3 or 4 minutes or until garlic is a deep, golden color, stirring frequently to prevent burning.

3. Pour garlic mixture and reserved cooking liquid over spaghetti, and toss to coat. Season with pepper, and garnish with parsley (if using).

PINCH OF SAGE

Watch the garlic carefully as it cooks because it's quick to burn. If you manage to burn the garlic every time, stir ¼ teaspoon water into the garlic before adding the olive oil to the skillet.

Splash of Lemon Asparagus

Steamed asparagus with just a splash of lemon juice brings a bright, fresh flavor.

Yield:	Prep time:	Cook time:	Serving size:
24 spears	5 minutes	3 minutes	4 spears

Each serving has:		
15.4 calories	1.3 mg sodium	

24 spears asparagus	1 TB. fresh lemon juice

1. Fill a steamer pot or a large saucepan with enough water to fall below the steamer basket when added, and bring to a boil over high heat. Add asparagus spears to a steamer basket, and place the basket in the pot or saucepan. Cover and steam asparagus over gently boiling water, reducing heat as necessary, for 3 to 5 minutes or until just tender-crisp.

2. Remove asparagus to a serving platter. Drizzle lemon juice over all.

PINCH OF SAGE

Forego the tedious task of peeling the skin off the bottom of each asparagus spear. Simply snap off and discard the bottom of each spear. Asparagus spears have a natural breaking point.

Wild and Brown Rice Pecan Dish

The toasted, nutty flavor of this simple rice medley pairs perfectly with just about any entrée.

Yield:	Prep time:	Cook time:	Serving size:
4 cups	4 minutes	61 minutes	½ cup
Each serving has:			
149.1 calories	2 mg sodium		

½ cup chopped unsalted pecans

1 TB. unsalted butter

½ cup uncooked brown rice

½ cup uncooked wild rice

¼ cup diced yellow onions

2 TB. chopped fresh parsley

1 TB. chopped fresh basil

¼ tsp. ground ginger

¼ tsp. Salt-Shaker Substitute (recipe in Chapter 14) or other salt-free salt substitute seasoning blend

¼ tsp. freshly ground black pepper

2 cups water

1. In a large skillet over medium heat, *toast* pecans for 5 minutes or until fragrant and toasted, shaking often to prevent burning. Remove pecans from the skillet.

2. In the same skillet, melt ½ tablespoon butter. Stir in brown rice and wild rice, and toast for 3 minutes or until golden, stirring often. Remove rice from the skillet.

3. Add remaining ½ tablespoon butter to the skillet, and melt. Add onions, parsley, basil, ginger, Salt-Shaker Substitute, and pepper. Cook for 3 minutes or until onions are golden, stirring frequently. Turn off heat. Return pecans and rice to the skillet, and stir to combine.

4. Preheat the oven to 350°F. Coat a 1½-quart baking dish with nonstick cooking spray.

5. Turn rice mixture into the prepared baking dish. Pour in water, and stir. Cover and bake for 50 to 55 minutes or until liquid is absorbed and rice is tender. Fluff with a fork before serving.

DEFINITION

Toast is a directive to heat a food, such as a bread, nut, spice, or grain, until it is fragrant and/or lightly browned to draw out its flavor and/or to crisp it. Closely watch any food you're toasting to prevent burning.

Basil-Tarragon Sautéed Mushrooms

Hearty mushroom slices are sizzled in a buttery, herb-heavy sauce.

Yield:	Prep time:	Cook time:	Serving size:
1⅓ cups	2 minutes	5 minutes	⅓ cup
Each serving has:			
39.3 calories	2.5 mg sodium		

1 TB. Herb-Flecked Butter (recipe in Chapter 14)

1 (8-oz.) pkg. sliced button mushrooms

1. In a medium nonstick skillet over medium heat, melt Herb-Flecked Butter.

2. Add mushrooms, and sauté for 4 or 5 minutes or until tender.

Salternative: You may substitute sliced baby portobello mushrooms if you prefer their meatier taste.

PINCH OF SAGE

Crimini? Baby portobellos? It's simply a marketing game. Portobello mushrooms are the mature form of crimini mushrooms. As portobello mushrooms grew in popularity, manufacturers began marketing crimini mushrooms as baby portobello mushrooms, sometimes with a higher price tag.

Green Beans Almondine

Buttery green beans complement the crunch of toasted almond slices.

Yield:	Prep time:	Cook time:	Serving size:
3 cups	10 minutes	10 minutes	½ cup
Each serving has:			
63.1 calories	3 mg sodium		

1 (16-oz.) pkg. frozen French-style green beans

1 TB. unsalted butter

¼ cup sliced unsalted almonds, toasted

1. Prepare green beans according to the package directions. Drain.

2. Stir butter into green beans until melted. Stir in almonds until evenly distributed. Serve immediately.

PINCH OF SAGE

To toast almonds, put them in a dry skillet over medium heat for 2 to 5 minutes. Watch the almonds carefully and shake often because they can be quick to burn.

Roasted Potatoes with Basil

Herbed butter sauce flavors the smoky roasted goodness of waxy new potatoes.

Yield:	Prep time:	Cook time:	Serving size:
12 potatoes	10 minutes	30 minutes	3 potatoes
Each serving has:			
123.3 calories	3.5 mg sodium		

1 lb. tiny new potatoes (*B size*)

2 TB. unsalted butter, melted

¼ tsp. freshly ground black pepper

2 TB. chopped fresh basil

1. Preheat the oven to 450°F.

2. Scrub new potatoes and place in a small casserole dish.

3. In a small bowl, stir together melted butter, pepper, and basil. Drizzle seasoned butter over new potatoes. Cover and bake for 30 minutes or until fork-tender.

Salternative: Feel free to substitute your favorite herb for the basil.

> **DEFINITION**
>
> **B size** potatoes are 1½ to 2¼ inches in diameter. You'll likely find them in a loose bin in the produce section.

Fruited Couscous

Savory couscous is sweetened with dried apricots and raisins plus the added crunch of almonds.

Yield:	Prep time:	Cook time:	Serving size:
3 cups	10 minutes	8 minutes	½ cup
Each serving has:			
155.50 calories	3.8 mg sodium		

1 cup sliced baby portobello (or crimini) mushrooms

½ medium yellow onion, diced

¾ cup uncooked whole-wheat couscous

¼ cup chopped dried apricots

¼ cup dark raisins

¼ cup chopped fresh parsley

1½ cups water

¼ cup chopped unsalted almonds

1. In a medium saucepan over high heat, combine mushrooms, onion, couscous, apricots, raisins, parsley, and water. Stir and bring to a boil. Reduce heat to low, cover, and simmer for 6 to 8 minutes or until fruit is tender and liquid is absorbed.

2. Stir in almonds until evenly distributed.

Salternative: Change the taste of this side dish by substituting dried cranberries for the apricots or pine nuts for the almonds.

PINCH OF SAGE

Although couscous is a coarsely ground pasta, it's often sold alongside grains and used as you would a grain. Couscous has long been a staple in North African cooking, where it's used much like rice. If you can't find whole-wheat couscous, simply substitute regular couscous in this recipe.

Tex-Mex Rice

Fresh tomato salsa pairs with nutty brown rice for a super-simple hot dish to accompany any south-of-the-border meal.

Yield:	Prep time:	Cook time:	Serving size:
3 cups	2 minutes	7 minutes	½ cup

Each serving has:			
82.3 calories	4.6 mg sodium		

2 cups cooked long-grain brown rice	1 cup Fresh-Taste Tomato Salsa (recipe in Chapter 13) or other low-sodium tomato salsa

1. In a medium saucepan over medium heat, combine rice and Fresh-Taste Tomato Salsa.

2. Cook, stirring occasionally, for 7 to 10 minutes or until heated through.

PINCH OF SAGE

Regular long-grain brown rice has a long cooking time, but you can find sodium-free packages. Cook a large batch when you have the time to save on the bit of sodium in quick-cooking instant rices (5 to 20 milligrams per serving). Store extra cooked rice in the freezer until you need it.

Simple Caraway Noodles

Buttery egg noodles hold the sweet, tangy flavor of caraway seeds.

Yield:	Prep time:	Cook time:	Serving size:
4 cups	5 minutes	10 minutes	1 cup
Each serving has:			
144.2 calories	5 mg sodium		

3 cups uncooked wide egg noodles
2 TB. unsalted butter

1 tsp. caraway seeds

1. Cook egg noodles according to the package directions (omit salt). Drain, and return to the pan.

2. Add butter, and stir until melted.

3. Add caraway seeds, and stir until evenly distributed.

Salternative: Add more caraway seeds if you like their distinctive sweet, tangy flavor.

Roasted Butternut Squash

Sweet winter squash carries a hot-sweet spiciness with deep, roasted flavor.

Yield:	Prep time:	Cook time:	Serving size:
4 cups	15 minutes	30 minutes	½ cup
Each serving has:			
70.2 calories	5.1 mg sodium		

1 medium (about 2-lb.) butternut
   squash
1½ TB. extra-virgin olive oil
⅜ tsp. crushed red pepper flakes or
   to taste

⅜ tsp. ground cinnamon
⅛ tsp. ground nutmeg

1. Preheat the oven to 400°F.

2. With a large, sharp knife, cut butternut squash in half lengthwise. Using a spoon, scoop out and discard strings and seeds. Using a vegetable peeler, peel butternut squash and wash under running water. Cut into 1-inch cubes.

3. On a large nonstick baking sheet, combine butternut squash cubes, extra-virgin olive oil, crushed red pepper flakes, cinnamon, and nutmeg. Stir to coat evenly, and arrange in a single layer. Bake for 30 minutes or until tender, stirring halfway through the baking time.

PINCH OF SAGE

Instead of discarding the seeds of the butternut squash (or any other winter squash), you can clean and roast them as you would pumpkin seeds.

Fettuccini with Basil-Almond Pesto

The classic basil and olive oil sauce is made with hearty toasted almonds and served over wide noodles.

Yield:	Prep time:	Cook time:	Serving size:
8 servings	20 minutes	10 minutes	1 ounce pasta with 1 tablespoon pesto

Each serving has:		
169.8 calories	6.5 mg sodium	

8 oz. fettuccini pasta	2 TB. sliced unsalted almonds, toasted
1 cup packed fresh basil leaves	¼ cup extra-virgin olive oil
1 TB. packed fresh parsley leaves	1 TB. finely grated Parmesan cheese
1 medium clove garlic, minced	

1. Cook pasta according to the package directions (omit salt). Lightly drain.

2. Place basil and parsley in a food processor, and pulse until chopped. Add garlic and almonds, and pulse until finely chopped. Pour in extra-virgin olive oil, and process for 20 seconds or until smooth, scraping down the sides as necessary.

3. Spoon mixture into a small bowl, and stir in Parmesan cheese.

4. Add pesto to pasta, and toss to coat. Serve warm or at room temperature.

PINCH OF SAGE

To refrigerate the pesto sauce, directly press plastic wrap onto the surface to prevent discoloration. You'll need to use the pesto within a few days.

Tomato-Studded Sugar Snap Peas

Sautéed in olive oil until crisp-tender, these sweet sugar snap peas are studded with tomato and onion.

Yield:	Prep time:	Cook time:	Serving size:
2 cups	15 minutes	5 minutes	½ cup
Each serving has:			
73.5 calories	10.7 mg sodium		

2 tsp. extra-virgin olive oil

½ tsp. garlic powder

2 cups fresh sugar snap peas, rinsed and trimmed

½ cup diced tomatoes (about 1 medium)

¼ cup diced yellow onions

1. In a small skillet over medium heat, heat extra-virgin olive oil. Stir in garlic powder, and cook for 30 seconds or just until golden.

2. Add sugar snap peas to the skillet, and sauté for 2 to 4 minutes or until nearing desired tenderness.

3. Add tomatoes and onions to the skillet, and sauté for 2 minutes or until onions are translucent.

Salternative: If fresh sugar snap peas are unavailable, you can substitute frozen sugar snap peas that have been thawed and drained. Cook in the skillet until heated through.

Lo Mein Noodles with Stir-Fried Vegetables

The deep flavor of sesame oil and bright cilantro season classic Asian-style veggies and lo mein noodles with the kick of a Serrano chili.

Yield:	Prep time:	Cook time:	Serving size:
6 servings	15 minutes	6 minutes	1 ounce noodles with ⅓ cup vegetables

Each serving has:	
177.7 calories	11.5 mg sodium

6 oz. lo mein noodles

2½ TB. sesame oil

⅔ cup trimmed Chinese snow peas

4 medium green onions, trimmed and sliced

1 medium red serrano chili pepper, ribs and seeds removed, and thinly sliced

½ cup julienned carrots

1 (8-oz.) can sliced water chestnuts, drained and rinsed

2 TB. chopped fresh cilantro

1. Cook lo mein noodles according to the package directions (omit salt). Rinse and drain well. Toss noodles with 1½ tablespoons sesame oil.

2. Heat remaining 1 tablespoon sesame oil in a wok or a large skillet over high heat. Add snow peas, green onions, serrano chili pepper, carrots, and water chestnuts, and stir-fry for 3 minutes or until vegetables are crisp-tender. Remove from heat, and stir in cilantro.

3. Serve stir-fried vegetables over noodles.

Salternative: You can substitute a less fiery chili pepper for the serrano pepper if you prefer.

 PINCH OF SAGE

To remove some of the chili pepper's heat, thoroughly cut away the chili pepper's ribs and discard all the seeds. This will make the dish more enjoyable for those who aren't fire-eaters.

Walnut-Apricot Dressing

This savory brown-rice-and-nut stuffing blend is sweetened with apricot and cinnamon.

Yield:	Prep time:	Cook time:	Serving size:
8 cups	5 minutes	30 minutes	½ cup

Each serving has:		
195.5 calories	16 mg sodium	

1½ cups dried apricots, cut in half	⅔ cup chopped unsalted walnuts
5 TB. unsalted butter	⅓ cup toasted sesame seeds
1⅓ cups diced yellow onions	1 heaping tsp. ground cinnamon
2 medium ribs celery, diced	¼ tsp. freshly ground black pepper
5 cups cooked long-grain brown rice	

1. In a small bowl, soak apricots in enough cool water to cover for 30 minutes. Drain well.

2. Meanwhile, preheat the oven to 350°F. Spray a 13×9×2-inch baking dish with non-stick cooking spray.

3. In a large skillet over medium heat, melt butter. Add onions and celery, and sauté for 5 to 7 minutes or until softened.

4. In the prepared baking dish, combine brown rice, onion mixture, and apricots. Add walnuts, sesame seeds, cinnamon, and pepper, and stir to combine thoroughly. Bake for 30 to 35 minutes or until top is golden.

PINCH OF SAGE

Remember to cook the rice without the optional salt and butter often called for in the package directions.

Indian-Curried Cauliflower

A creamy curry sauce flavors these steamed cauliflower florets.

Yield:	Prep time:	Cook time:	Serving size:
8 cups	10 minutes	8 minutes	1 cup

Each serving has:	
22.8 calories	26 mg sodium

1 medium head cauliflower, cut into medium florets	1 TB. fresh lime juice
¼ cup fat-free plain yogurt	1½ to 2 tsp. salt-free curry powder or to taste

1. Fill a steamer pot or a large saucepan with enough water to fall below the steamer basket when added, and bring to a boil over high heat. Add cauliflower florets to a steamer basket, and place the basket in the pot or saucepan. Cover and steam cauliflower over gently boiling water, reducing heat as necessary, for 8 minutes or until just crisp-tender. Remove cauliflower to a serving dish.

2. In a small bowl, stir together yogurt, lime juice, and curry powder until well blended. Pour over cauliflower, and stir until evenly coated.

PINCH OF SAGE

When seasoning with curry powder, add a small amount at first and then add more to your taste. Curry powder can have a strong flavor if you're not used to it. You can always add more as needed—but you can't take it out if you added too much!

Dilly Carrots Almondine

A buttery sauce seasons crisp-tender baby carrots topped with crunchy almonds.

Yield:	Prep time:	Cook time:	Serving size:
1½ cups	5 minutes	15 minutes	½ cup
Each serving has:			
94.9 calories	40.8 mg sodium		

½ lb. baby carrots (about 1½ cups)	2 TB. sliced unsalted almonds
½ cup water	½ tsp. dried dill weed
1 TB. unsalted butter	Scant ½ tsp. ground nutmeg

1. In a small saucepan over medium-high heat, boil carrots in water for 10 minutes or until tender-crisp. Drain and set aside.

2. In the same saucepan over low heat, melt butter. Stir in almonds, dill weed, and nutmeg, and cook for 1 or 2 minutes.

3. Return carrots to the saucepan, stir until evenly coated, and serve immediately.

Salternative: You can substitute fresh dill for the dried variety, but remember you need to use more fresh to equal the same flavor of using dry. In this recipe, use ½ tablespoon chopped fresh dill, adjusting to taste.

Quick Cowboy Corn Fritters

Savory fritters serve up sweet corn with bits of green onions and red bell peppers.

Yield:	Prep time:	Cook time:	Serving size:
18 fritters	10 minutes	12 minutes	2 fritters
Each serving has:			
114.9 calories	79.4 mg sodium		

1 (15.25-oz.) can unsalted whole-kernel corn, drained	½ medium red bell pepper, ribs and seeds removed, and diced
1 large egg, beaten	¼ cup whole-wheat flour
2 medium green onions, tops sliced and white parts diced	¼ cup extra-light olive oil

1. In a medium bowl, combine corn, egg, green onions, red bell pepper, and whole-wheat flour. Stir until well mixed.

2. In a medium skillet over medium heat, heat extra-light olive oil. When hot, spoon in corn mixture to make 18 (2-inch) fritters, frying in batches. Fry for 2 minutes or until golden brown. Turn and fry for 2 more minutes or until golden brown on underside. Remove with a slotted spoon to a paper towel–lined plate to drain.

Salternative: A 15.25-ounce can of whole-kernel corn equals 1¾ cups when drained. You can use the equivalent of thawed and drained frozen corn for this recipe if you like.

Mediterranean Millet

Tender eggplant, creamy cannellini beans, tomatoes, and basil flavor mild millet for whole-grain goodness.

Yield:	Prep time:	Cook time:	Serving size:
5 cups	10 minutes	25 minutes	½ cup

Each serving has:	
107.8 calories	219 mg sodium

4 dry-packed sun-dried tomatoes

½ cup hot water

2 TB. extra-virgin olive oil

1 medium yellow onion, finely diced

½ small eggplant, diced

2 medium cloves garlic, crushed

1 (14.5-oz.) can no-salt-added diced tomatoes, with juice

1½ cups cooked whole millet

½ tsp. dried basil

⅛ tsp. freshly ground black pepper

1 (15-oz.) can no-salt-added cannellini beans, rinsed and drained

1. In a small bowl, soak sun-dried tomatoes in hot water until softened. Chop tomatoes.

2. In a large, deep skillet over medium-low heat, heat extra-virgin olive oil. Add onion and eggplant, and sauté for 10 minutes or until tender.

3. Add garlic, and stir in diced tomatoes. Simmer for 10 to 15 minutes.

4. Add millet, basil, sun-dried tomatoes, soaking water, pepper, and cannellini beans to the skillet. Stir to combine, and heat through.

Sweet Treats and Sippers

Finding sodium-appropriate desserts and other sweets can be a challenge because salt and other high-sodium products are perennial ingredients in baked goods and beverages. But with a few helpful substitutions and low-sodium ingredients, you can delight in delectable drinks, yummy cookies, scrumptious brownies and fudges, creamy sauces and puddings, luscious cakes, rich cheesecakes, tasty pies and tarts, and mouthwatering crisps and cobblers.

We have used unsalted butter in preparing the following treats because it's widely available and always sodium free. If you need to watch your saturated fat and cholesterol intake, you can choose to substitute a sodium-sensible margarine. Just keep in mind that any baked good should be prepared with a margarine that contains at least 60 percent fat. Spreads lower in fat cannot be used for baking purposes.

The Cookie Jar

In This Chapter

- Bypassing salty, store-bought cookies
- Baking mouthwatering low-sodium cookies
- Making the most of sodium-free ingredients

If you're missing a favorite treat of milk and cookies because you're following a new low-sodium diet, cheer up! Cookies, in moderation, can be incorporated into a sodium-restricted diet. You just need a low-sodium recipe, or you can prepare a much-loved recipe using sodium-wise leavening agents.

Even low-sodium cookies are treats, though, and you'll still need to control your urge to eat until they're gone. The upside is that you'll keep your cookie jar full longer.

In the Cookie Aisle

A trip down your supermarket's cookie aisle may surprise you. Most of those yummy cookies in pretty packages are packed with sodium.

If you find it hard to believe that a cookie is salty, try a taste test. After you've weaned yourself off a heavily salted diet and are eating at your personal sodium-responsible point, get one of those cookies you crave. You may want to have a glass of water nearby because trust us—packaged cookies will taste salty to you now.

A Batch of Solutions

Of course, if you like to bake, you can whip up a low-sodium cookie recipe anytime you're feeling like a certain furry, blue monster (who happens to be improving his diet now, too—a lot like you). And if you don't enjoy baking cookies from scratch, you can purchase a low-sodium cookie mix. Really though, mixing up the dough for a simple cookie may be easier than getting your hands on a special low-sodium packaged mix.

The recipes in this chapter give you a collection of cookies to bake that don't require special sodium-free leavening agents. If you have a collection of favorite cookie recipes you just don't want to give up, you can give sodium-free baking powder, sodium-free baking soda, and low-sodium cream of tartar products a try. Having a stash of suitable baking products to use in place of traditional high-sodium baking ingredients allows you to bake many of your favorite recipes. (For more information on special leavening agents, see Chapter 2.)

Just remember that even cutting out much of the sodium doesn't give you free reign to devour the whole batch. Cookies are still hefty deliverers of saturated fat and calories. Be aware of the serving size of 1 or 2 cookies.

One reason you'll need to watch your portions is the amount of unsalted butter called for in these recipes. The butter keeps these unleavened treats soft and palatable. If your doctor or nutritionist has suggested a sodium-sensible margarine, please follow that recommendation.

SALT PITFALL

Low-fat margarine spreads can't be used for baking. If you substitute margarine for unsalted butter in these cookie recipes, you'll need one with at least 60 percent fat.

Russian Tea Cakes

Simple cookie bites are flavored with nutty pecan pieces and sweetened with a topping of confectioners' sugar.

Yield:	Prep time:	Chill time:	Cook time:	Serving size:
3 dozen cookies	20 minutes	2 hours	24 minutes	1 cookie

Each serving has:				
86.7 calories	0 mg sodium			

1 cup (2 sticks) unsalted butter, softened	1 tsp. pure vanilla extract
$\frac{1}{4}$ cup plus 3 TB. confectioners' sugar	2 cups all-purpose flour
	$\frac{1}{2}$ cup unsalted chopped pecans, toasted

1. In a large bowl, combine butter, $\frac{1}{4}$ cup confectioners' sugar, and vanilla extract. Using an electric mixer on medium speed, mix for 3 minutes or until well blended, scraping down the sides of the bowl as needed.

2. Mix in flour and pecans for 2 or 3 minutes or until dough forms. Cover and chill dough for 2 hours.

3. Preheat the oven to 375°F. Coat cookie sheets with nonstick cooking spray.

4. Roll dough into 36 (1-inch) balls, and place on the prepared cookie sheets 2 inches apart. Bake for 8 to 10 minutes or until just lightly browned. Let stand on the cookie sheet for 1 minute before removing to a wire rack to cool.

5. Place remaining 3 tablespoons confectioners' sugar on a sheet of waxed paper. Roll tops of cookies in confectioners' sugar, shaking off excess. Store cookies in an airtight container, separating layers with waxed paper.

PINCH OF SAGE

If you've forgotten to set out the butter at room temperature to soften, you can accomplish it quickly in the microwave—if you're careful. Place the butter in a small, microwave-safe bowl and cover with waxed paper. Cook on defrost power for 15-second intervals just until the butter is softened, being careful not to let it melt.

Sugared Cinnamon Sticks

These stick-shape cookies are lightly sweetened with cinnamon and sugar.

Yield:	Prep time:	Cook time:	Serving size:
3½ dozen cookies	25 minutes	22 minutes	2 cookies

Each serving has:	
126.5 calories	0.1 mg sodium

1 cup (2 sticks) unsalted butter, softened	3 TB. granulated sugar
1 tsp. pure almond extract	2 cups all-purpose flour
1 TB. ground cinnamon	

1. Preheat the oven to 300°F. Lightly coat cookie sheets with nonstick cooking spray with flour.

2. In a medium bowl, combine butter, almond extract, cinnamon, 2 tablespoons sugar, and flour. Using a pastry blender, 2 knives, or your fingers, cut in butter until dough forms and cleans the sides of the bowl.

3. Roll dough into ropes ½ inch in diameter. Cut into 42 (2-inch) sections, and arrange sections on the prepared cookie sheets, spacing slightly. Bake for 22 to 25 minutes or just until cookies are colored.

4. Remove cookies to a wire rack to cool slightly. Sprinkle remaining 1 tablespoon sugar over tops of cookies. Cool completely before storing in an airtight container.

PINCH OF SAGE

For less mess, place a sheet of waxed paper under the wire rack. After sprinkling the cookies with sugar, fold up the waxed paper and toss it.

Pistachio-Studded Lime Cookies

The cornmeal base with undertones of cardamom is topped with a sweet lime glaze speckled with creamy pistachio pieces.

Yield:	Prep time:	Freeze time:	Cook time:	Serving size:
3 dozen cookies	40 minutes	1 hour	27 minutes	1 cookie

Each serving has:		
122.1 calories	0.6 mg sodium	

1 cup (2 sticks) unsalted butter, softened

¾ cup granulated sugar

2 large egg yolks

1 TB. plus 5 tsp. fresh lime juice

3 tsp. grated lime zest

1½ cups all-purpose flour

1 cup yellow cornmeal

½ tsp. ground cardamom

1½ cups confectioners' sugar

1 TB. water

2 drops green food coloring

⅓ cup chopped unsalted pistachios

1. In a large mixing bowl, and using an electric mixer on medium speed, beat butter and sugar for 2 minutes or until light and fluffy, scraping down the sides of the bowl as needed.

2. Add egg yolks, 1 tablespoon lime juice, and 2 teaspoons lime zest, and beat for 1 minute or until well blended, scraping down side of bowl as needed.

3. In a medium bowl, stir together flour, cornmeal, and cardamom until blended. Add to the mixing bowl, beating on low speed until dough forms.

4. Divide dough in half and place on sheets of waxed paper. Form each half into a 10-inch log, and wrap in waxed paper. Freeze dough for 1 hour or until firm.

5. Preheat the oven to 350°F.

6. Unwrap logs, and cut dough into slices. Arrange slices 1 inch apart on nonstick cookie sheets. Bake for 9 to 11 minutes or until edges are golden. Let stand on cookie sheet for 1 minute before removing to a wire rack to cool completely.

7. Meanwhile, in a medium bowl, combine confectioners' sugar, remaining 5 teaspoons lime juice, remaining 1 teaspoon lime zest, water, and green food coloring. Stir until smooth. Spread over tops of cooled cookies, and sprinkle pistachios over wet icing. Let stand until set. Store in an airtight container, separating layers with waxed paper.

PINCH OF SAGE

You can make-ahead the cookie dough and store it, well wrapped, in the freezer for up to 1 month. When you're ready to serve the cookies, allow the frozen logs to stand at room temperature for about 10 minutes before slicing.

Shortbread Jam Thumbprints

Mild almond cookies feature the sweetness of raspberries and a sugary glaze.

Yield:	Prep time:	Freeze time:	Serving size:
4 dozen cookies	35 minutes	24 minutes	2 cookies
Each serving has:			
142.1 calories	0.7 mg sodium		

⅔ cup granulated sugar

1 cup (2 sticks) unsalted butter, softened

1¼ tsp. pure almond extract

2 cups all-purpose flour

¼ cup seedless red raspberry spreadable fruit or your favorite spreadable fruit

½ cup confectioners' sugar

1½ tsp. water

1. Preheat the oven to 350°F.

2. In a large mixing bowl, combine sugar, butter, and ½ teaspoon almond extract. Using an electric mixer on medium speed, beat for 2 or 3 minutes or until light and fluffy, scraping down the sides of the bowl as needed.

3. Reduce speed to low, add flour, and beat for 2 or 3 minutes or until well mixed and dough forms.

4. Shape dough into 48 (1-inch) balls, and place on ungreased cookie sheets 2 inches apart. Using your thumb, make an indentation in the center of each cookie. (Small cracks may form; gently push any large cracks back together.) Fill each indentation with ¼ teaspoon red raspberry spreadable fruit.

5. Bake for 12 to 14 minutes or until edges of cookies are golden. Let stand for 1 minute on the cookie sheets. Remove cookies to a wire rack set over a sheet of waxed paper to cool.

6. Meanwhile, in a small bowl, combine confectioners' sugar, remaining ¾ teaspoon almond extract, and water. Whisk together until smooth. Drizzle in a thin stream over tops of cookies, and allow glaze to set. Store in an airtight container, separating layers with waxed paper.

PINCH OF SAGE

If you have a rounded ½-teaspoon measuring spoon, you can use it to make the indentations in the cookies. The pockets will be more uniform and help keep the spreadable fruit from oozing onto your cookie sheets.

Simply Scottish Shortbread Cookies

The classic sweet dough is lightly flavored with almond and sprinkled with sugar.

Yield:	Prep time:	Freeze time:	Serving size:
2 dozen cookies	15 minutes	1 hour	1 (2¼×1½-inch) cookie
Each serving has:			
125.1 calories	1 mg sodium		

1 cup (2 sticks) unsalted butter, softened

½ cup plus 2 tsp. granulated sugar

1 tsp. almond extract

2 cups all-purpose flour

1. Preheat the oven to 300°F. Coat a 9×9×2-inch baking dish with nonstick cooking spray.

2. In a large bowl, combine butter, ½ cup sugar, and almond extract. Using an electric mixer on medium-low speed, cream for 8 minutes or until fluffy. Beat in flour, ½ cup at a time.

3. Evenly press dough into the prepared pan. With the tines of a fork, prick surface of dough all over. Bake for 1 hour or until top is golden brown.

4. Remove from the oven, and immediately sprinkle remaining 2 teaspoons sugar evenly over top. *Score* dough into 2¼×1½-inch squares, and cool completely in the pan on a wire rack. Store any leftovers in an airtight container.

DEFINITION

Score directs the cook to make shallow, incomplete cuts into a food. Here, scoring the soft dough allows for cutting the cookies after they've cooled without crumbling.

Peppermint Candy–Sprinkled Cookies

These cornstarch-heavy cookies are infused with peppermint and glazed with crunchy candies.

Yield:	Prep time:	Chill time:	Cook time:	Serving size:
39 cookies	30 minutes	30 minutes	36 minutes	2 cookies

Each serving has:	
84.8 calories	1.1 mg sodium

1¼ cups confectioners' sugar	1¼ cups all-purpose flour
1 cup (2 sticks) plus 1 TB. unsalted butter, softened	½ cup cornstarch
1½ tsp. pure vanilla extract	2 TB. fat-free milk
¼ tsp. pure peppermint extract	10 hard peppermint candies, finely crushed

1. In a large bowl, combine ½ cup confectioners' sugar, 1 cup butter, vanilla extract, and peppermint extract. Using an electric mixer on medium speed, beat for 2 or 3 minutes or until well mixed.

2. Reduce speed to low, add flour and cornstarch, and beat for 3 or 4 minutes or until thoroughly blended. Cover and chill dough for 30 minutes.

3. Preheat the oven to 350°F.

4. Form dough into 39 (1-inch) balls, and place 2 inches apart on nonstick cookie sheets. Bake for 12 or 13 minutes or just until edges are lightly browned. Let cookies stand on cookie sheets for 2 minutes before gently removing to a wire rack placed over waxed paper to cool.

5. Meanwhile, in a small bowl, combine remaining ¾ cup confectioners' sugar, remaining 1 tablespoon butter, and milk. Whisk until smooth, and spread over tops of cookies. Sprinkle crushed peppermint candies over top, and let set before storing in an airtight container, separating layers with waxed paper.

PINCH OF SAGE

The peppermint candies topping these delicate cookies needs to be finely crushed. To crush the hard peppermint candies, unwrap and place them in a zipper-lock bag. Pound them into fine pieces using a rolling pin or the flat side of a meat mallet.

Classic No-Bake Cookies

A jumble of cocoa-flavored oats and pecans are the simple answer to a sweets craving.

Yield:	Prep time:	Cook time:	Serving size:
3½ dozen cookies	20 minutes	5 minutes	2 cookies

Each serving has:			
212.6 calories	3.8 mg sodium		

2 cups granulated sugar	3 cups quick oats
½ cup fat-free milk	¾ cup chopped unsalted pecans
4 TB. unsalted butter	1 tsp. pure vanilla extract
2 TB. cocoa powder	

1. In a large, heavy saucepan over high heat, combine sugar, milk, butter, and cocoa powder, and bring to a boil, stirring constantly. Boil and stir for 2 minutes. Remove from heat.

2. Stir in oats, pecans, and vanilla extract until thoroughly combined.

3. Working quickly and carefully, drop mixture from a tablespoon onto the waxed paper. Cool until set.

PINCH OF SAGE

Precisely measuring the dry ingredients (not overmeasuring) and working quickly while the mixture is hot lends to the success of this recipe. If the mixture cools too much before you finish forming the cookies, you can reheat the mixture over low heat—but you may lose some cookies to the pan.

Almond Macaroons

Simple almond flavor is served up in a soft cookie.

Yield:	Prep time:	Cook time:	Serving size:
32 cookies	25 minutes	30 minutes	1 cookie

Each serving has:		
63.7 calories	4.1 mg sodium	

1 (8-oz.) can almond paste	2 large egg whites
1¼ cups granulated sugar	

1. Preheat the oven to 325°F. Line cookie sheets with parchment paper.

2. Cut almond paste into small pieces, and place in a large bowl. Add sugar. Using an electric mixer on low speed, beat for 15 minutes or until fine crumbs form. Add egg whites, and mix until dough forms.

3. Using a small cookie scoop or tablespoon, drop dough onto the prepared cookie sheets 1 inch apart. Bake for 15 to 17 minutes or until golden. Cool completely on cookie sheets on wire racks. Peel cookies off the parchment paper, and store in an airtight container.

PINCH OF SAGE

You can store unused egg yolks in the refrigerator in a covered container with a little added water for a day or two.

Sweet Maple Cookies

These maple and brown sugar–flavored cookies tempt serious sweet tooths with their super-sweet bite.

Yield:	Prep time:	Cook time:	Serving size:
6 dozen cookies	15 minutes	36 minutes	1 cookie
Each serving has:			
63.6 calories	4.5 mg sodium		

2⅓ cups firmly packed light brown sugar

1 cup (2 sticks) unsalted butter, softened

2 large eggs, at room temperature

1 tsp. pure vanilla extract

½ tsp. pure maple extract

2 cups all-purpose flour

1. Preheat the oven to 375°F.

2. In a large bowl, combine light brown sugar, butter, eggs, vanilla extract, and maple extract. Using an electric mixer on medium speed, mix for 2 or 3 minutes or until well blended, scraping down the sides of the bowl as needed.

3. Stir in flour by hand until incorporated and dough cleans the sides of the bowl.

4. Using a small cookie scoop or tablespoon, drop dough onto nonstick cookie sheets 2 inches apart. Bake for 6 to 8 minutes or until just golden around the edges. Let stand on the cookie sheets for 1 or 2 minutes before removing to wire racks to cool completely. Store in an airtight container.

PINCH OF SAGE

If you can't find pure maple extract for these super-sweet cookies, you can substitute imitation maple extract.

Golden Lemon Ribbons

The lemon tang shines through in these light, puffed cookies.

Yield:	Prep time:	Chill time:	Cook time:	Serving size:
4 dozen cookies	30 minutes	3 hours	10 minutes	2 ribbons

Each serving has:	
84.8 calories	5.9 mg sodium

½ cup confectioners' sugar

4 TB. unsalted butter, softened

2 large eggs, at room temperature

2 large egg yolks, at room temperature

2 tsp. grated lemon zest

1 TB. fresh lemon juice

2 cups all-purpose flour

Canola oil

1. In a small mixing bowl, combine confectioners' sugar, butter, eggs, and egg yolks. Using an electric mixer on medium speed, beat for 2 or 3 minutes until blended, scraping down the sides of the bowl as needed. Stir in lemon zest and lemon juice.

2. Pour flour into a medium bowl. Stir in lemon mixture until blended and dough forms. Cover and chill for 3 hours.

3. On a lightly floured work surface, roll out dough to a ¼-inch thickness. Using a sharp knife, cut dough into ¾×2½-inch strips. Cut a slash down the center of each strip, and pull one end through the opening. (Strips should resemble a knotless bow tie.)

4. Heat 1 inch canola oil in an electric skillet to 375°F. Add ribbons in batches, and fry until they float and are golden. Remove with a slotted spoon to a paper towel–lined plate, and drain well. Serve warm or at room temperature. Store in an airtight container.

PINCH OF SAGE

If you need to chill the dough for more than 3 hours, let the dough stand at room temperature for a few minutes before rolling it out to make it more workable.

Brownies, Bars, and Fudges

In This Chapter

- Sodium-responsible sweets—from scratch
- Avoiding the sodium in prepackaged mixes
- Spotting high-sodium ingredients
- Delicious dessert bites

Sweet treats are sometimes the perfect ending to a meal or a wonderful afternoon pleasure. You've perhaps discovered they can be too high in sodium. What to do? Make your own!

Brownies, bars, and fudges are simple enough to whip up. By making these bite-size desserts yourself, you can indulge a craving without ruining your resolve to stick to your low-sodium diet.

Thinking Outside the Box

Boxed brownie and dessert mixes boast homemade taste with the convenience of a single dry ingredient. One of the dry ingredients in that mix, though, is salt. Another is baking soda. Perhaps another is baking powder. Then, you'll add a couple eggs, and the sodium count is now too excessive for your needs. If you're a confirmed boxed-mix baker, you can find some low-sodium mixes to whip up.

But we'll let you in on a secret: baking from scratch can be just as easy. If you keep a few basic ingredients on hand—flour, cocoa powder, pure vanilla extract—you can stir up a brownie batter in just a few more measurements over a packaged mix.

Plus, making brownies and bars from your own scratch recipes allows you to substitute low-sodium ingredients:

- If your doctor or nutritionist has approved your use of a potassium chloride salt substitute, switch one intended for baking with the salt called for in a recipe.

- Sodium-free baking soda and baking powder can greatly reduce the sodium in a sweet treat.

- Replace any mayonnaise with fat-free plain yogurt.

- Trade regular peanut butter for natural peanut butter.

- If the milk chocolate called for in a recipe takes the sodium count too high, replace some or all of it with semisweet or another type of chocolate.

- Use the unsalted variety for all nuts.

Substitute, substitute, substitute!

PINCH OF SAGE

A 6-ounce package (1 cup) milk chocolate chips contains 80 to 133 milligrams sodium. The same package of semisweet chocolate chips has only 18 milligrams sodium. Sodium-free semisweet chocolate chips are also available.

Itty, Bitty Bites

We all crave a little something sweet now and then. Just be careful that reducing the sodium count of your favorite treats doesn't lull you into believing you can wolf down the whole pan. Fat, cholesterol, and calories still count, so it's best to stick to the suggested serving size.

Super-Easy Peanut Butter Marble Fudge

Chocolate and peanut butter swirl their sweet flavors together in this creamy fudge.

Yield:	Prep time:	Cook time:	Serving size:
45 squares	15 minutes	1 hour	2 squares

Each serving has:		
149 calories	0.3 mg sodium	

2½ cups confectioners' sugar

2 TB. plus 2 tsp. cocoa powder

1 cup unsalted natural peanut butter, at room temperature

⅓ cup unsalted butter, melted

1½ tsp. pure vanilla extract

1. Coat a 9×5 pan. Chill for 1 hour or until firm. Cut into squares.

PINCH OF SAGE

This sweet treat makes a great gift for fudge lovers, and it's quick and easy to make. You can double the recipe, pressing the fudge into a 9×9 nonstick baking pan coated with nonstick cooking spray.

Mucho Mocha Brownies

The flavors of chocolate and coffee meld in these fluffy, moist brownies.

Yield:	Prep time:	Cook time:	Serving size:
16 brownies	22 minutes	20 minutes	1 (1¾×2¾-inch) brownie
Each serving has:			
208.7 calories	11.1 mg sodium		

1½ tsp. instant coffee granules	1 cup granulated sugar
½ cup hot water	½ cup (1 stick) unsalted butter
1 tsp. fresh lemon juice	2 TB. unsweetened cocoa powder
¼ cup fat-free milk	1 large egg, at room temperature
½ cup all-purpose flour	½ tsp. sodium-free baking soda
½ cup whole-wheat flour	½ tsp. vanilla extract

1. Preheat the oven to 400°F. Coat an 11×7-inch baking pan with nonstick cooking spray.

2. In a small bowl, dissolve coffee granules in hot water. Set aside.

3. In a measuring cup, pour lemon juice into milk. Set aside for 5 minutes to curdle.

4. In a large bowl, stir together all-purpose flour, whole-wheat flour, and sugar. Set aside.

5. In a small saucepan over medium heat, combine butter, coffee mixture, and cocoa powder. Bring to a boil, slowly stirring constantly. Remove from heat and continue stirring for 5 minutes to cool slightly.

6. Pour cocoa mixture over flour mixture, and stir until moistened. Add curdled milk and egg, and stir to mix. Add sodium-free baking soda and vanilla extract, and stir to blend.

7. Quickly turn batter into the prepared pan. Bake for 20 minutes or until a cake tester inserted in the center comes out clean. Cool in the pan on a wire rack before cutting to serve.

PINCH OF SAGE

To test an egg for freshness, fill a deep glass or other container with tap water. Carefully place the egg in the water. An easy rule to remember is "if it sinks, it's safe; if it floats, it's foul."

Chocolate-Nut Candy Squares

Toffee, chocolate, and walnuts delight the sweet tooth in this cool treat.

Yield:	Prep time:	Cook time:	Freeze time:	Serving size:
35 squares	10 minutes	15 minutes	2 hours	1 square

Each serving has:				
162.1 calories	9 mg sodium			

35 very-low-sodium saltine
   crackers (1 sleeve)

1 cup (2 sticks) unsalted butter

1 cup firmly packed light brown
   sugar

$1\frac{1}{2}$ cups semisweet chocolate chips

1 cup chopped unsalted walnuts

1. Preheat the oven to 400°F. Line a $14\frac{1}{4}\times9\frac{1}{4}\times1$-inch baking sheet with parchment paper.

2. Arrange crackers in a single layer on the prepared baking sheet.

3. In a medium saucepan over medium heat, melt butter and light brown sugar, and bring to a boil. Boil for 3 minutes, slowly stirring constantly to scrape the bottom of the pan. Pour butter mixture over crackers, and quickly spread to cover all as necessary. Bake for 5 minutes.

4. Evenly distribute chocolate chips over crackers. Bake for 2 minutes or just until chocolate chips are softened. Spread chocolate chips evenly over crackers.

5. Sprinkle walnuts over top, and press into chocolate.

6. Using a knife, score candy along edges of crackers. (Feel around a little if crackers have "floated" a bit.) Freeze the pan for at least 2 hours or until solid. Break along scored lines to serve. Store any leftovers in a sealable freezer bag in the freezer.

 PINCH OF SAGE

The crackers will fit exactly on the baking sheet in a 5×7-cracker rectangle. If your crackers aren't fitting, first try turning them the other direction. (Saltine crackers aren't precisely square.) If you can't get the crackers to fit, it's important to fill the baking sheet in a single layer—even if you have to use partial crackers along the edges.

Bleached Blondies

A brownie without chocolate—a.k.a. a blondie—lets the simple baked-good vanilla flavor come through.

Yield:	Prep time:	Cook time:	Serving size:
1 dozen blondies	10 minutes	25 minutes	1 blondie
Each serving has:			
181.3 calories	10.7 mg sodium		

1 cup all-purpose flour	2 large eggs, at room temperature
1 cup granulated sugar	1 tsp. pure vanilla extract
½ cup (1 stick) unsalted butter, softened	

1. Preheat the oven to 350°F. Coat an 8×8×2-inch baking pan with nonstick cooking spray with flour.

2. In a large bowl, combine flour, sugar, butter, eggs, and vanilla extract. Using an electric mixer on medium speed, beat for 3 minutes or until well blended.

3. Spread batter evenly in the prepared pan. Bake for 25 to 30 minutes or until golden and a cake tester inserted in the center comes out clean. Cool in the pan on a wire rack. Cut into bars to serve.

Salternative: You can fold ¼ cup chopped unsalted walnuts or pecans into the batter if you like.

PINCH OF SAGE

Blondies are good snacks for people who can't have chocolate. They're really just brownies without the chocolate flavoring.

Chocolate-Chocolate-Chip Brownies

Classic brownies get even more chocolaty with the addition of miniature chocolate chips.

Yield:	Prep time:	Cook time:	Serving size:
1 dozen brownies	15 minutes	25 minutes	1 brownie

Each serving has:		
208.7 calories	11.1 mg sodium	

1 cup all-purpose flour	2 large eggs, at room temperature
¼ cup cocoa powder	1 tsp. pure vanilla extract
1 cup granulated sugar	¼ cup miniature semisweet
½ cup (1 stick) unsalted butter, softened	chocolate chips

1. Preheat the oven to 350°F. Coat an 8×8×2-inch baking pan with nonstick cooking spray with flour.

2. In a large bowl, combine flour, cocoa powder, sugar, butter, eggs, and vanilla extract. Using an electric mixer on medium speed, beat for 3 minutes or until well blended. Fold in chocolate chips.

3. Spread batter in the prepared pan. Bake for 25 minutes or until brownies test done. Cool in the pan on a wire rack. Cut into bars to serve.

Salternative: Substitute chopped unsalted walnuts for the chocolate chips, if you prefer.

PINCH OF SAGE

Cocoa powder is a good way to satisfy your chocolate cravings. It has only 1 milligram sodium in a tablespoon. Plus, it has no saturated fat, no cholesterol, and only 12 calories per tablespoon.

Micro-Quick Chocolate Fudge

These smooth, sweet chocolaty fudge squares are studded with crunchy walnuts.

Yield:	Prep time:	Cook time:	Chill time:	Serving size:
64 squares	15 minutes	3 minutes	3 hours	2 squares

Each serving has:	
170 calories	11.4 mg sodium

½ cup dark corn syrup

⅓ cup fat-free evaporated milk

3 cups semisweet chocolate chips

¾ cup confectioners' sugar

2 tsp. pure vanilla extract

1½ cups chopped unsalted walnuts

1. Line an 8×8×2-inch pan with plastic wrap.

2. In a 3-quart microwave-safe dish, combine dark corn syrup and evaporated milk, stirring with a wooden spoon to blend well. Cook on high for 3 minutes or until boiling well. Remove from the microwave.

3. Quickly stir in chocolate chips until melted and mixture is blended. Quickly add confectioners' sugar, vanilla extract, and walnuts, stirring until blended. Beat mixture with the wooden spoon for 1 or 2 minutes or until thick and glossy.

4. Turn mixture into the prepared pan, and spread evenly. Chill for 3 hours or until firm. Cut into squares to serve. Store leftovers in the refrigerator.

PINCH OF SAGE

Having your ingredients premeasured helps you add them quickly and confidently to the heated mixture.

Toasted Fruity Granola Bars

Nutty, fruit-filled oat bars taste toasty and sweet.

Yield:	Prep time:	Cook time:	Serving size:
24 bars	15 minutes	35 minutes	1 bar
Each serving has:			
230.2 calories	12.7 mg sodium		

3½ cups rolled oats

½ cup sesame seeds

½ cup chopped almonds

¾ cup unsalted butter

½ cup firmly packed light brown sugar

½ cup honey

½ tsp. ground nutmeg

½ cup chopped dried apricots

½ cup golden raisins

½ cup sweetened flaked coconut

1. Preheat the oven to 350°F.

2. In a 10×15-inch nonstick baking pan, combine oats, sesame seeds, and almonds. Bake for 15 minutes or until almonds are lightly browned, stirring every 5 minutes.

3. Meanwhile, in a large saucepan over low heat, melt butter. Remove from heat, and stir in light brown sugar, honey, and nutmeg. Add oat mixture, apricots, raisins, and coconut, and stir until evenly coated.

4. Coat the 10×15-inch baking pan with nonstick cooking spray with flour. Turn mixture into the prepared pan, and press in evenly. Bake for 20 minutes or until browned and bubbling in the center. Cool on a wire rack for 20 minutes before cutting into bars. Cool completely before storing in an airtight container.

Salternative: You can grease and flour the baking pan by hand if you don't have nonstick cooking spray with flour. The pan will be hot from the oven, though! For safety, prepare another 10×15-inch baking pan for baking the bars.

PINCH OF SAGE

If you buy your sesame seeds already toasted, just add them to the oat mixture after removing the baking pan from the oven following step 1. No need to toast them a second time.

Golden Sunshine Bars

A tender pastry crust serves up a sweet orange filling.

Yield:	Prep time:	Cook time:	Serving size:
20 bars	10 minutes	55 minutes	1 bar
Each serving has:			
197.9 calories	13.2 mg sodium		

$\frac{1}{2}$ cup plus 2 tsp. confectioners' sugar

$2\frac{1}{4}$ cups all-purpose flour

1 cup (2 sticks) unsalted butter, softened

4 large eggs, beaten

1 cup granulated sugar

6 TB. fresh orange juice

1. Preheat the oven to 300°F.

2. In a large bowl, combine $\frac{1}{2}$ cup confectioners' sugar and 2 cups flour. Using a pastry blender, 2 knives, or your fingertips, cut in butter until coarse crumbs form. Using your fingers, press crust mixture into a 13×9×2-inch baking pan. Bake for 30 minutes or until edges are just golden.

3. In a large bowl, combine eggs, granulated sugar, orange juice, and remaining $\frac{1}{4}$ cup flour. Using an electric mixer on medium speed, beat for 2 or 3 minutes or until well blended. Pour egg mixture over hot crust, and bake for 25 to 30 minutes or until set.

4. Sprinkle remaining 2 teaspoons confectioners' sugar over top, and cut into bars while still warm.

PINCH OF SAGE

The orange filling for these bars won't appear done, but instead still wet and glossy. You need to test the dryness with your fingertip.

Walnut-Studded Chocolate Sponge Bars

This chocolaty, nutty bar bakes up with a tender, spongy texture.

Yield:	Prep time:	Cook time:	Serving size:
12 bars	15 minutes	22 minutes	1 bar

Each serving has:		
133.5 calories	13.6 mg sodium	

¾ cup all-purpose flour	1 large egg, at room temperature
¼ cup cocoa powder	½ cup fat-free sour cream
½ cup granulated sugar	¼ cup water
¼ cup miniature semisweet chocolate chips	1 tsp. pure vanilla extract
¼ cup unsalted chopped walnuts	12 unsalted walnut halves

1. Preheat the oven to 325°F. Coat an 8×8×2-inch baking dish with nonstick cooking spray with flour.

2. In a large bowl, combine flour, cocoa powder, and sugar, and stir until blended. Stir in chocolate chips and walnuts. Make a well in the center of dry ingredients.

3. In a small bowl, beat egg. Whisk in sour cream, water, and vanilla extract until blended.

4. Pour wet ingredients into well in dry ingredients, and fold in dry ingredients just until moistened.

5. Gently spread batter into the prepared dish. Evenly space walnut halves across top of batter. Bake for 22 minutes or until edges are firm and center is just set. Remove to a wire rack to cool. Cut into bars.

PINCH OF SAGE

Use a light hand when you fold together the ingredients. You don't want to overmix this batter. The bars will go from spongy to rubbery if you do.

Lemony Cloud Bars

A flaky pastry crust supports a tangy-sweet lemon topping.

Yield:	Prep time:	Chill time:	Serving size:
16 bars	35 minutes	47 minutes	1 bar
Each serving has:			
164.2 calories	16 mg sodium		

⅓ cup plus ¼ cup unsalted butter	2 large eggs, separated
¼ cup confectioners' sugar	1 TB. grated lemon zest
1¼ cups all-purpose flour	¼ cup fresh lemon juice
1 cup granulated sugar	1 cup fat-free milk

1. Preheat the oven to 350°F.

2. In a large bowl, blend ⅓ cup butter with confectioners' sugar. Mix in 1 cup flour until fine crumbs form. Using your fingers, press mixture into the bottom of an ungreased 9×9×2-inch nonstick baking pan. Set aside.

3. In the same large bowl, combine remaining ¼ cup butter, granulated sugar, and remaining ¼ cup flour. Using an electric mixer on medium speed, mix for 10 minutes or until well combined and packing firm around the edge of the bowl if not scraped.

4. Beat in egg yolks, lemon zest, and lemon juice. Blend in milk. Set aside.

5. Bake crust for 12 minutes or until golden around edges.

6. Meanwhile, in a small bowl, and using the electric mixer with clean, dry beaters on high speed, beat egg whites until soft peaks form. Fold egg whites into lemon mixture until well combined. (Do not blend or stir.)

7. Pour topping over hot crust, and bake for 35 to 40 minutes or until top is a deep golden brown. Cool in the pan on a wire rack. Cut into bars, and refrigerate any leftovers.

SALT PITFALL

Take care when separating your eggs. The whites won't peak if you've gotten even a drop of yolk in them.

Chocolate-Crusted Pecan Bars

Creamy, sweetened pecans rest atop a cocoa-crusted pastry base.

Yield:	Prep time:	Cook time:	Serving size:
24 bars	30 minutes	35 minutes	1 bar

Each serving has:		
214.7 calories	20.4 mg sodium	

1¼ cups all-purpose flour

1 cup confectioners' sugar

½ cup cocoa powder

1 cup (2 sticks) unsalted butter, softened

1 (14-oz.) can fat-free sweetened condensed milk

1 large egg, at room temperature

2 tsp. pure vanilla extract

1½ cups unsalted chopped pecans

1. Preheat the oven to 350°F. Coat a 13×9×2-inch baking pan with nonstick cooking spray with flour.

2. In a large bowl, stir together flour, confectioners' sugar, and cocoa powder. Using a pastry blender, 2 knives, or your fingertips, cut in butter until mixture is crumbly. Using your fingers, press evenly into the bottom of the prepared pan. Bake for 15 minutes.

3. Meanwhile, in a medium bowl, combine sweetened condensed milk, egg, and vanilla extract. Using an electric mixer on medium speed, beat for 2 minutes or until blended. Stir in pecans.

4. Spread evenly over crust. Bake for 20 to 25 minutes or until topping is set. Cool on a wire rack. Cut into bars to serve.

PINCH OF SAGE

If you're looking to reduce the cholesterol in recipes, replace the called-for egg with an egg substitute.

Sweet Endings

In This Chapter

- Creating low-sodium cakes
- Indulging in cheesecake
- Perfectly sodium-sensible pies
- Fruity crisps and cobblers

What's dinner without dessert? Maybe you know the answer to this question because your doctor or nutritionist has warned you away from your favorite baked dessert dishes, and now your sweet tooth feels neglected.

The recipes in this chapter can cheer up both you and your sweet tooth. As long as you make helpful substitutions and maintain an appropriate portion, you can happily dig in to desserts again. Go grab your fork!

A Piece of Cake

Whether the occasion is a birthday, a wedding, a baby shower, a graduation, or some other special milestone, we celebrate with cake. Made with traditional baking ingredients, a cake is a bit high in sodium. However, you can bake your own low-sodium cakes using sodium-free baking substitutes. (For more information on sodium-free baking products, see Chapter 2.)

Not a from-scratch baker? You can choose from several low-sodium cake mixes, as well as frosting mixes, to whip up a "homemade" cake from a box. But give the cake recipes in this chapter a try. We hope you'll find them as delicious as we do.

Say "Cheesecake!"

Cream cheese—the creamy, cheesy ingredient that gives a cheesecake the taste and texture that melts on your tongue—contains at least 80-some milligrams sodium per 1-ounce serving. (The number jumps up dramatically when the cream cheese is fat-free.) Each block of cream cheese is 8 ounces; some cheesecake recipes call for as many as 4 blocks! You don't have to be an ace at math to know the resulting number of milligrams sodium is perilous. And that's not including any of the sodium added in from the graham cracker crust, sour cream, or eggs. What's a cheesecake connoisseur to do?

Give the two cheesecake variations in this chapter a try. You may find a low-sodium alternative you like. Otherwise, you'll just have to save up all your sodium budget to blow on a teensy, tiny sliver of your favorite.

My Sweetie Pie (or Sweet Tart)

Not all pies and tarts are created equal. Fruit pies and tarts are likely to be more reasonable, sodium-wise, than mile-high cream pies. Plus, preparing the dessert yourself allows you to cut any salt from the crust recipe.

If you like your pie with a slice of cheddar cheese or a scoop of ice cream, choose low-sodium products. You don't want to bake a special low-sodium pie only to top it with high-sodium additions.

> **PINCH OF SAGE**
>
> Get into the habit of cutting your 9-inch pies and tarts into 8 slices instead of just 6. You'll benefit by less sodium, fewer calories, and less fat in the smaller pieces.

Crisps and Cobblers

Crisps are good dessert choices for those on a sodium-restricted diet. Typical ingredients are reasonable in sodium, if not sodium free. Cobblers may require some rising agent, so be certain to substitute a sodium-free baking product as needed.

An important pitfall to avoid when choosing crisps and cobblers for dessert is piling them high with sodium-dense additions. If you like your crisps and cobblers served with frozen yogurt, ice cream, or whipped cream, keep an eye on the serving size of both the crisp or cobbler and the topping. The topping's going to provide some additional sodium, so be sure to tally up the total for the entire dessert.

Perfect Piecrust

Tender and pleasantly flaky, this crust is the perfect complement for all your dessert pies.

Yield:	Prep time:	Serving size:
1 (9-inch) piecrust	15 minutes	$\frac{1}{8}$ crust

Each serving has:		
137.5 calories	0.1 mg sodium	

6 TB. trans-fat-free shortening   5 TB. cold water
1 cup all-purpose flour

1. In a medium bowl, and using a pastry blender, 2 knives, or your fingertips, cut shortening into flour until crumbly. Add cold water, 1 tablespoon at a time, stirring with a fork until dough forms and cleans the sides of the bowl.

2. Turn out dough onto a lightly floured work surface, and roll out to an 11-inch circle. Fold circle into quarters, and transfer to a 9-inch nonstick pie pan. Place point of dough in the center of the pan and unfold and press dough into the pan. With a sharp knife, trim edge of dough as needed. Flute or crimp edge as desired.

3. Follow desired pie recipe to fill and bake.

SALT PITFALL

Use only the amount of water needed to form a dough, which may be more or less than the amount called for.

Spiced Zucchini Cobbler

Nicely spiced with a crumbly, tender crust and topping, the zucchini will pleasantly surprise your apple-cobbler fans.

Yield:	Prep time:	Cook time:	Serving size:
9 servings	25 minutes	51 minutes	3×3-inch portion

Each serving has:			
371.1 calories	2.2 mg sodium		

4 cups peeled and chopped zucchini	1 tsp. ground cinnamon
⅓ cup fresh lemon juice	¼ tsp. ground nutmeg
1½ cups granulated sugar	2 cups all-purpose flour
	¾ cup (1½ sticks) unsalted butter

1. In a medium saucepan over medium heat, combine zucchini and lemon juice. Cook, stirring occasionally, for 15 to 20 minutes or until zucchini is tender.

2. Stir in ½ cup sugar, ½ teaspoon cinnamon, and nutmeg. Cook for 1 minute, and remove from heat.

3. Preheat the oven to 375°F. Grease a 9×9×2-inch baking dish with nonstick cooking spray with flour.

4. In a large bowl, stir together flour and remaining 1 cup sugar. Using a pastry blender, 2 knives, or your fingertips, cut in butter until crumbly.

5. Stir ¼ cup flour mixture into zucchini mixture. Turn ½ remaining flour mixture into the prepared dish, and press in using your fingers. Spread zucchini mixture over top. Sprinkle remaining flour mixture over zucchini mixture. Sprinkle remaining ½ teaspoon cinnamon over top. Bake for 35 minutes or until top is browned. Cool on a wire rack. Serve warm or cold.

PINCH OF SAGE

This recipe is a great way to use up your bountiful zucchini harvest—or your neighbor's. Serve it as you would an apple cobbler.

Crunchy Oat Crust

Nutty and crunchy, this substantial crust holds up to full-flavored fillings.

Yield:	Prep time:	Cook time:	Serving size:
1 (9-inch) piecrust	10 minutes	10 minutes	$\frac{1}{8}$ crust

Each serving has:			
186 calories	3.1 mg sodium		

1 cup quick oats

$\frac{1}{3}$ cup chopped unsalted pecans

$\frac{1}{4}$ cup firmly packed light brown sugar

4 TB. unsalted butter, melted

1. Preheat the oven to 350°F.

2. In a medium bowl, stir together oats, pecans, and light brown sugar. Drizzle in butter, and stir with a fork until evenly moistened.

3. Turn mixture into a nonstick 9-inch pie pan. Press evenly onto the bottom and up the sides of the pan to form a crust. Bake for 10 minutes or until lightly browned and set. Cool on a wire rack before filling as desired.

Salternative: You can use your favorite chopped unsalted nuts for this piecrust, such as walnuts, peanuts, or almonds.

PINCH OF SAGE

Brown sugar is sold in light and dark varieties. The designations refer to the color produced by the amount of added molasses. If you only have dark brown sugar available, you can substitute $\frac{2}{3}$ cup dark brown sugar plus $\frac{1}{3}$ cup granulated sugar for 1 cup light brown sugar.

Pilgrim's Cranberry-Apple Crisp

A buttery, crunchy, nutty, crisped topping coats tender, sweet-tart apples and cranberries.

Yield:	Prep time:	Cook time:	Serving size:
8 servings	20 minutes	45 minutes	3½×2¾-inch portion
Each serving has:			
468.4 calories	6.2 mg sodium		

1½ cups quick oats

½ cup plus 3 TB. all-purpose flour

½ cup firmly packed light brown sugar

¼ cup chopped unsalted pecans

½ cup (1 stick) unsalted butter, melted

3 cups peeled and chopped Golden Delicious apples

2 cups cranberries, fresh or frozen

1 cup granulated sugar

1. Preheat the oven to 350°F. Grease an 11×7×2-inch nonstick baking pan with non-stick cooking spray with flour.

2. In a medium bowl, combine oats, ½ cup flour, light brown sugar, and pecans. Stir. Drizzle in melted butter, and stir until well combined. Set aside.

3. In another medium bowl, combine apples, cranberries, sugar, and remaining 3 tablespoons flour. Stir to coat, and turn into the prepared pan. Sprinkle oat mixture over top. Bake for 45 to 50 minutes or until top is browned and fruit is tender.

PINCH OF SAGE

If you're using frozen cranberries, add them right to the mixture frozen. You don't need to thaw them before using.

Strawberry Double Crisp

Sweet strawberry slices are bedded between layers of nutty, crunchy goodness.

Yield:	Prep time:	Cook time:	Serving size:
6 servings	20 minutes	40 minutes	4×2½-inch square
Each serving has:			
375.2 calories	8.4 mg sodium		

3 cups sliced fresh strawberries

⅓ cup granulated sugar

⅔ cup quick oats

⅔ cup whole-wheat flour

½ cup firmly packed light brown sugar

¼ cup chopped unsalted pecans

5 TB. unsalted butter

1. Preheat the oven to 350°F. Spray the bottom of an 8×8×2-inch baking dish with nonstick cooking spray.

2. In a medium bowl, place strawberries. Sprinkle sugar over top. Set aside.

3. In a medium bowl, stir together oats, whole-wheat flour, light brown sugar, and pecans. Using a pastry blender, 2 knives, or your fingertips, cut in butter until crumbly and evenly distributed.

4. Spread 2 cups oat mixture over the bottom of the prepared dish. Stir strawberry mixture, pour into the dish, and spread remaining oat mixture over top. Bake for 40 minutes or until browned and bubbly. Serve warm or chilled.

SALT PITFALL

If you scoop on vanilla frozen yogurt or ice cream to this or any of the desserts in this chapter, that adds sodium. Don't forget to calculate the additional sodium the "extras" add.

Bubbly Blueberry Crisp

With a tasty, crumbly topping, lightly spiced blueberries shine through in this crisp.

Yield:	Prep time:	Cook time:	Serving size:
6 servings	20 minutes	25 minutes	4×2½-inch portion
Each serving has:			
330.4 calories	11.7 mg sodium		

3 cups fresh blueberries

1 TB. fresh lemon juice

½ cup granulated sugar

¼ tsp. ground cinnamon

¼ tsp. ground nutmeg

¾ cup all-purpose flour

½ cup firmly packed light brown sugar

6 TB. unsalted butter, at room temperature

1. Preheat the oven to 350°F.

2. In a large bowl, combine blueberries, lemon juice, sugar, cinnamon, and nutmeg. Stir to coat evenly. Turn into an 8×8×2-inch nonstick baking pan.

3. In another large bowl, combine flour and light brown sugar. Using a pastry blender, 2 knives, or your fingertips, cut in butter until crumbly. Evenly sprinkle over top of blueberry mixture. Bake for 25 minutes or until bubbly and golden brown. Serve warm or cold, as desired.

SALT PITFALL

Is your brown sugar usually rock hard? Avoid this by storing it in the refrigerator in a tightly sealed container.

Topsy-Turvy Peach Cobbler

Tender dough rises to envelop summer-fresh peach slices in this sweet cobbler.

Yield:	Prep time:	Cook time:	Serving size:
6 servings	15 minutes	55 minutes	4½×3-inch piece
Each serving has:			
273.5 calories	17.7 mg sodium		

4 TB. unsalted butter

1 cup all-purpose flour

2 tsp. sodium-free baking powder

¾ cup granulated sugar

¾ cup fat-free milk

2 cups peeled and sliced fresh peaches (about 1 lb. or 4 medium peaches)

1. Preheat the oven to 325°F.

2. Place butter in a 9×9×2-inch nonstick baking pan, and melt in the preheating oven.

3. Meanwhile, in a medium bowl, stir together flour, baking powder, and sugar. Pour in milk, and stir until blended. Pour batter into the prepared pan over bubbly butter.

4. Arrange peaches over batter without touching the edges of the pan. Do not mix. Bake for 55 to 60 minutes or until top is browned. Serve warm or cold with frozen yogurt, ice cream, or whipped cream, as desired.

PINCH OF SAGE

To peel peaches, place them in a bowl and pour boiling water over them. Let the peaches stand for 1 minute and then plunge them into ice water. The skins should remove easily.

Honey Vanilla Cupcakes with Buttercream Icing

Tender, dense cupcakes are filled with honey flavor and iced with sweet vanilla creaminess.

Yield:	Prep time:	Cook time:	Serving size:
1 dozen cupcakes	30 minutes	20 minutes	1 cupcake
Each serving has:			
332.5 calories	19.1 mg sodium		

½ cup plus 6 TB. unsalted butter, softened

½ cup granulated sugar

2 large eggs, at room temperature

½ cup plus 1½ TB. fat-free milk

½ cup honey

1½ cups all-purpose flour

2¾ tsp. vanilla extract

1¾ tsp. sodium-free baking powder

1½ cups confectioners' sugar

1. Preheat the oven to 350°F. Line a 12-cup nonstick muffin pan with paper cupcake liners.

2. In a large bowl, and using an electric stand mixer on medium-low speed, *cream* ½ cup butter and granulated sugar for 8 minutes or until light and fluffy. Add eggs, 1 at a time, and beat very well after each addition (about 2 minutes).

3. In a measuring cup, combine ½ cup milk and honey. Stir until well blended. (Let stand mixer run while stirring mixture for 1 or 2 minutes.)

4. Alternately beat flour and then milk mixture into creamed mixture, starting with and ending with flour. (We had 3 flour additions and 2 milk mixture additions.)

5. Stop the mixer, and stir in 2 teaspoons vanilla extract until blended. Stir in baking powder until thoroughly incorporated. (Batter will have a whipped topping–like consistency.)

6. Immediately spoon batter into the prepared cups, filling ⅞ full. Bake for 20 to 25 minutes or until a cake tester or a wooden toothpick inserted in the center of a cupcake comes out clean. Cool in the pan on a wire rack for 10 minutes. Remove and cool completely on the wire rack before icing.

7. While cupcakes cool, in a small mixing bowl, and using the mixer on medium-low speed, cream remaining 6 tablespoons butter and confectioners' sugar for 5 minutes or until light and fluffy. Add remaining 1½ tablespoons milk and remaining ¾ teaspoons vanilla extract, and beat until blended.

8. Ice each cooled cupcake with about 2 tablespoons icing. Store any leftover cupcakes in the refrigerator.

DEFINITION

Cream refers to beating a fat such as butter, often with another ingredient such as sugar, to soften and aerate a batter. Creaming butter with sugar should result in a smooth, light, pale mixture that no longer feels of the graininess of sugar.

No-Bake Cherry Vanilla Pie

Light and creamy vanilla-flavored filling surrounds sweet-tart cherries in a nutty, crunchy crust.

Yield:	Prep time:	Chill time:	Serving size:
1 (9-inch) pie	10 minutes	2 hours	1 slice ($\frac{1}{8}$ pie)
Each serving has:			
267.6 calories	20.3 mg sodium		

1 (6-oz.) container fat-free, sugar-free cherry-vanilla yogurt

1 cup French vanilla frozen whipped topping, thawed

1 (15-oz.) can pitted cherries, well drained

1 Crunchy Oat Crust (recipe earlier in this chapter)

1. In a medium bowl, stir together yogurt and whipped topping. Stir in cherries.

2. Turn mixture into Crunchy Oat Crust. Chill for at least 2 hours before serving.

Salternative: Substitute plain whipped topping if French vanilla isn't available.

PINCH OF SAGE

Experiment and create your own favorite version of this easy-to-make pie by using different whipped topping flavors, yogurt flavors, and fruit.

Sweet and Creamy Strawberry Swoops

Succulent strawberries pair with a brown-sugar-and-cinnamon-sweetened sour cream.

Yield:	Prep time:	Chill time:	Serving size:
½ cup dip with 32 strawberries	5 minutes	1 hour	2 tablespoons dip with 8 strawberries

Each serving has:		
85 calories	25.8 mg sodium	

½ cup fat-free sour cream

1 TB. firmly packed light brown sugar

Pinch ground cinnamon

32 large whole strawberries, rinsed

1. In a small bowl, stir together sour cream, light brown sugar, and cinnamon until well combined.

2. Cover and chill for at least 1 hour before serving.

3. Hull strawberries as desired, and serve with dip.

Salternative: For a large gathering, you can double this recipe, using ⅛ teaspoon cinnamon to 1 cup sour cream. You can even double it again, if needed.

SALT PITFALL

Choose your fat-free or reduced-fat sour creams carefully. Many manufacturers add sodium as they reduce fat. Compare the nutrition labels closely. We've found Breakstone's or Knudsen's fat-free sour cream has just 25 milligrams sodium per 2 tablespoon serving.

Golden Lemon Pound Cake

This dense, tender pound cake is a lemon lover's dream for flavor and pretty presentation.

Yield:	Prep time:	Cook time:	Serving size:
1 fluted tube cake ring	35 minutes	1¼ hours	1 slice (1/12 cake)
Each serving has:			
546.8 calories	28.4 mg sodium		

1½ cups (3 sticks) unsalted butter, softened

3 cups granulated sugar

5 large eggs, at room temperature

3 cups all-purpose flour

2 TB. pure lemon extract

¾ cup lemon-lime soda

1. Preheat the oven to 325°F. Spray a 12-cup fluted tube pan with nonstick cooking spray with flour.

2. In a large bowl, and using an electric mixer on medium speed, blend butter and sugar for 20 minutes or until thoroughly combined and very creamy.

3. Add eggs, 1 at a time, beating well after each addition. Add flour and lemon extract, and beat until incorporated. Gently fold in lemon-lime soda until blended.

4. Pour batter into the prepared pan. Bake for 1¼ hours or until a cake tester inserted in the center comes out clean. Cool in the pan on a wire rack for 20 minutes. Turn out cake onto the wire rack to cool completely.

PINCH OF SAGE

Preheating the oven is especially important when baking baked goods, and particularly essential if you're not using the traditional sodium-laden leavening agents. Baked goods must be exposed to the proper temperature at the very start of baking for the leavening process to occur properly.

Cake-Crusted Lemon Custard Pie

You'll love this smooth, tangy-sweet, lemon custard in a tender flaky crust.

Yield:	Prep time:	Cook time:	Serving size:
1 (9-inch) pie	25 minutes	40 minutes	1 slice (⅛ pie)
Each serving has:			
260.7 calories	32 mg sodium		

1 Perfect Piecrust (recipe earlier in this chapter)

2 large eggs, at room temperature, separated

1 TB. unsalted butter, softened

2 TB. all-purpose flour

¾ cup granulated sugar

¼ cup fresh lemon juice

1 cup fat-free milk

1. Preheat the oven to 350°F.

2. With the tines of a fork, prick the bottom and sides of Perfect Piecrust. Bake for 5 minutes.

3. Meanwhile, in a small bowl, and using an electric mixer on medium speed, beat egg whites until frothy. Increase speed to high, and beat until stiff peaks form. Set aside.

4. In a large bowl, and using an electric mixer on medium speed, beat butter and flour until fine crumbs form. Add sugar, egg yolks, lemon juice, and milk, and beat until well blended. Fold in egg whites.

5. Pour mixture into partially baked piecrust. Bake for 35 minutes or until top is browned and filling is set. Remove to a wire rack to cool. Serve at room temperature or cold.

PINCH OF SAGE

To enjoy this lemony pudding without the piecrust, try our Cake-Crusted Lemon Pudding (recipe in Chapter 25).

Harvest Pumpkin Pie

Pure pumpkin purée is fluffed up with sweetened and spiced whipping cream and served in a tender piecrust.

Yield:	Prep time:	Cook time:	Serving size:
1 (9-inch) pie	10 minutes	1 hour	1 slice (⅛ pie)

Each serving has:		
322 calories	34.4 mg sodium	

2 large eggs, at room temperature	1 (15-oz.) can solid-pack pumpkin (not pumpkin pie filling)
1 cup firmly packed light brown sugar	1 tsp. pumpkin pie spice
½ cup light whipping cream	1 Perfect Piecrust (recipe earlier in this chapter)

1. Preheat the oven to 425°F.

2. In a large bowl, and using an electric mixer on medium speed, beat eggs for 3 minutes or until thick and lemon-colored. Add light brown sugar, whipping cream, pumpkin, and pumpkin pie spice. Beat for 1 or 2 minutes or until well blended.

3. Pour pumpkin mixture into Perfect Piecrust. Bake for 10 minutes.

4. Reduce the oven temperature to 350°F. Bake for 50 minutes or until a knife inserted in the center comes out clean. Cool completely on a wire rack before cutting.

PINCH OF SAGE

If the edge of your piecrust is browning too quickly while the pie cooks, you can use a pie shield to protect it from overbrowning. Covering the edge of the crust with aluminum foil works, too.

Decadent Chocolate-Orange Cake

Serve this dense, chocolaty cake topped with orange-flavored whipped cream when dessert is the main attraction.

Yield:	Prep time:	Cook time:	Chill time:	Serving size:
1 (9-inch) round cake	55 minutes	50 minutes	8 hours	1 slice ($\frac{1}{12}$ cake)

Each serving has:	
503 calories	56.2 mg sodium

1$\frac{2}{3}$ cups semisweet chocolate chips	$\frac{1}{2}$ cup light whipping cream
1 tsp. instant coffee granules	2 TB. grated orange zest
10 large eggs, separated	$\frac{1}{4}$ tsp. fresh orange juice
1$\frac{1}{4}$ cups unsalted butter, softened	$\frac{1}{4}$ tsp. pure vanilla extract
1$\frac{1}{4}$ cups plus 2 TB. granulated sugar	

1. Preheat the oven to 350°F. Grease a 9-inch springform pan with nonstick cooking spray with flour.

2. In a small saucepan over lowest heat, melt chocolate chips with coffee granules, stirring until smooth. Cool.

3. In a large bowl, and using an electric mixer on medium speed, beat egg whites until frothy. Increase speed to high, and beat until stiff peaks form. Set aside.

4. In another large bowl, and using the mixer on medium speed, blend butter and 1$\frac{1}{4}$ cups sugar for 2 minutes or until light and fluffy.

5. Add chocolate mixture, and beat until blended. Add egg yolks, 1 at a time, and beat well after each addition. Beat for 15 minutes, and fold in egg whites until blended.

6. Pour batter into the prepared pan. Bake for 50 minutes or until a cake tester inserted in the center comes out clean. Cool completely in the pan on a wire rack. Cover and chill for at least 8 hours.

7. Meanwhile, in a small, chilled mixing bowl, combine whipping cream, orange zest, remaining 2 tablespoons sugar, orange juice, and vanilla extract. With chilled beaters, beat on medium speed for 3 or 4 minutes or until soft peaks form.

8. Remove cake from the pan, and frost on the top and side, or chill frosting until time to frost cake. Cover and chill cake if not serving immediately.

PINCH OF SAGE

Chill the beaters and small mixing bowl by placing them in the refrigerator before mixing the frosting. When your ingredients, bowl, and beaters are cold, your whipped cream will remain stable for several hours after beating.

Rainbow Fruit Tart

The buttery crust carries a sweet filling bursting with fresh, juicy fruits.

Yield:	Prep time:	Cook time:	Serving size:
1 (9-inch) tart	30 minutes	45 minutes	1 slice (⅛ tart)

Each serving has:			
207.4 calories	59.7 mg sodium		

⅓ cup unsalted butter, softened

1¼ cups all-purpose flour

5 TB. ice water

1 cup egg substitute

⅓ cup granulated sugar

1 tsp. pure almond extract or pure vanilla extract

¼ cup fat-free milk

1 cup mixed fruit (sliced peaches; peeled, halved, and sliced kiwifruit; sliced bananas; mandarin orange segments; crushed pineapple; or other fruits)

1. Preheat the oven to 350°F.

2. In a medium bowl, and using a pastry blender, 2 knives, or your fingertips, cut butter into flour until mixture is crumbly. Add ice water, 1 tablespoon at a time, stirring with a fork until dough forms and cleans the sides of the bowl.

3. Turn out dough onto a lightly floured work surface, and roll out to an 11-inch circle. Fold circle into quarters, and transfer to a 9-inch nonstick pie pan, placing point of dough in the center of the pan and unfolding and pressing dough into the pan. Make a ½-inch decorative flute around the edge.

4. In a medium bowl, combine egg substitute, sugar, and almond extract. Whisk to blend.

5. In a small saucepan over high heat, heat milk until bubbles form around edge of the pan. Gradually whisk milk into egg substitute mixture. Pour into crust. Bake for 45 minutes or until set. Cool completely on a wire rack, and cover and chill for 2 hours.

6. To serve, arrange mixed fruit decoratively on top of filling.

> **PINCH OF SAGE**
>
> If you choose fruits that will quickly discolor, such as apples or bananas, rub the cut surfaces with a little lemon juice to prevent browning.

Merry Berry Tart

A chocolaty crust complements the sweet, fresh berries it holds.

Yield:	Prep time:	Cook time:	Serving size:
1 (9-inch) tart	30 minutes	45 minutes	1 slice (⅛ tart)
Each serving has:			
207.6 calories	60.2 mg sodium		

1¼ cups all-purpose flour

2 TB. cocoa powder

⅓ cup unsalted butter, softened

5 TB. ice water

1 cup egg substitute

⅓ cup granulated sugar

1 tsp. pure vanilla extract

¼ cup fat-free milk

1 cup mixed berries (sliced strawberries, blueberries, red raspberries, and/or blackberries)

1. Preheat the oven to 350°F.

2. In a medium bowl, stir together flour and cocoa powder. Using a pastry blender, 2 knives, or your fingers, cut in butter until mixture is crumbly. Add ice water, 1 tablespoon at a time, stirring mixture with a fork until dough forms and cleans the sides of the bowl.

3. Turn out dough onto a work surface lightly dusted with cocoa powder, and roll out to an 11-inch circle. Fold circle into quarters, and transfer to a 9-inch nonstick pie pan, placing dough point in the center of the pan and unfolding and pressing dough into the pan. Make a ½-inch decorative flute around the edge.

4. In a medium bowl, combine egg substitute, sugar, and vanilla extract. Whisk to blend.

5. In a small saucepan over high heat, heat milk until bubbles form around edge of the pan. Gradually whisk milk into egg substitute mixture. Pour into crust. Bake for 45 minutes or until set. Cool completely on a wire rack, and cover and chill for 2 hours.

6. To serve, arrange mixed berries decoratively on top of filling.

PINCH OF SAGE

To easily flute the edge of the crust, trim any excess dough with a sharp knife, leaving about a 1 inch overhang around the rim. Fold the dough under itself, making it even with the edge of the pie pan. Place each thumb on either side of the crust edge. Crimp by pushing one thumb forward and the other thumb backward. Work your way around the edge, inserting one thumb into a previously made indentation and shaping a new notch with the other.

Yogurt-Baked Cheesecake

Try a slice of this airy, crustless, cheesecake-like dessert topped with traditional sweet-tart cherries.

Yield:	Prep time:	Cook time:	Chill time:	Serving size:
1 (9-inch) cheesecake	15 minutes	22 minutes	2 hours	1 slice ($\frac{1}{8}$ cheesecake)
Each serving has:				
91.3 calories	65.4 mg sodium			

3 egg whites, at room temperature

2 cups fat-free plain yogurt

3 TB. granulated sugar

1 tsp. pure vanilla extract

1 TB. fresh lemon juice

1 TB. cornstarch

1 cup cherry pie filling

1. Preheat the oven to 325°F.

2. In a small mixing bowl, and using an electric mixer on medium speed, beat egg whites until frothy. Increase speed to high, and beat until soft peaks form.

3. In a large bowl, combine yogurt, sugar, vanilla extract, lemon juice, and cornstarch. Mix until blended. Fold in egg whites.

4. Turn mixture into a 9-inch nonstick pie pan. Bake for 22 to 25 minutes or until top is golden. Cool on a wire rack, and chill for at least 2 hours before serving. Spoon 2 tablespoons cherry pie filling over each slice.

Salternative: Use the fruit topping of your choice for a prettier presentation with good taste. Try blueberry, strawberry, peach, or your favorite.

PINCH OF SAGE

Like a traditional cheesecake, this yogurt cheesecake will crack on the top. Covering it up with a fruit topping is a simple solution to hide the cracks.

Silky Tofu Cheesecake

In this creamy cheesecake with a traditional graham-cracker crust, silky tofu plays a starring role.

Yield:	Prep time:	Cook time:	Serving size:
1 (9-inch) cheesecake	25 minutes	45 minutes	1 slice ($\frac{1}{12}$ cheesecake)
Each serving has:			
171.3 calories	76.2 mg sodium		

$1\frac{1}{2}$ cups graham cracker crumbs

2 tsp. plus 1 cup granulated sugar

2 TB. water

1 TB. extra-light olive oil

1 (14-oz.) pkg. soft tofu, well drained and coarsely chopped

$\frac{1}{3}$ cup fat-free milk

1 large egg, at room temperature

1 TB. grated lemon zest

$\frac{1}{4}$ cup fresh lemon juice

3 TB. all-purpose flour

1. Preheat the oven to 350°F. Grease a 9-inch springform pan with nonstick cooking spray with flour.

2. In a medium bowl, combine graham cracker crumbs, 2 teaspoons sugar, water, and extra-light olive oil. Stir with a fork until evenly moistened. Pat onto the bottom and about $\frac{1}{2}$ inch up the sides of the prepared pan.

3. In a food processor, combine tofu, milk, egg, remaining 1 cup sugar, lemon zest, lemon juice, and flour. Purée for 30 seconds or until smooth. Pour filling into crust.

4. Place a pan of hot water on the bottom oven rack and cheesecake on the middle oven rack. Bake for 45 minutes or until just set in center. Remove the pan to a wire rack, and run a knife around the edge of the pan to loosen cheesecake. Cool completely, and cover and chill for at least 2 hours before serving. Top with cherry, blueberry, or strawberry pie filling as desired.

PINCH OF SAGE

When you're baking in a springform pan, set the pan on a baking sheet until you're sure it's not going to leak. If it starts to leak, bake with the sheet under the pan.

Lightweight Carrot Cake

This light, tender treat satisfies your desire for spiced carrot cake without a heavy slice topped with cream cheese frosting.

Yield:	Prep time:	Cook time:	Serving size:
16 pieces	25 minutes	30 minutes	1 (3¼×1¼-inch) piece
Each serving has:			
195.4 calories	105.2 mg sodium		

3 large eggs, separated

½ cup granulated sugar

⅔ cup fat-free milk

1 tsp. fresh lemon juice

1 cup cake flour

1 cup whole-wheat flour

1 cup firmly packed light brown sugar

1 tsp. sodium-free baking powder

1 tsp. sodium-free baking soda

1½ tsp. ground cinnamon

⅓ cup light olive oil

1½ cups grated carrots

1 TB. confectioners' sugar

1. Preheat the oven to 350°F. Grease a 13×9×2-inch baking pan with nonstick cooking spray with flour.

2. In a small bowl, and using an electric mixer on medium speed, beat egg whites until frothy. Gradually add granulated sugar, increase speed to high, and beat until stiff.

3. In a measuring cup, measure milk. Stir in lemon juice and then let stand.

4. In a large bowl, combine cake flour, whole-wheat flour, light brown sugar, baking powder, baking soda, and cinnamon. Stir to blend.

5. Add olive oil and milk mixture, and mix well. Add egg yolks, and mix well. Fold in egg whites, and fold in carrots.

6. Turn batter into the prepared pan. Bake for 30 minutes or until a cake tester inserted in the center comes out clean. Cool on a wire rack. Sprinkle confectioners' sugar over top of cake just before serving.

> **PINCH OF SAGE**
>
> You can frost this carrot cake with a traditional cream cheese frosting, but remember that cream cheese is high in sodium, especially if you opt for the fat-free version to avoid the saturated fat and cholesterol of regular cream cheese.

Ooey-Gooey Puddings and Sauces

In This Chapter

- Easy-to-make puddings
- Sweet and rich lo-so sauces
- Toppings, coatings, and syrups for sodium-restricted desserts
- Employing ingredients with low sodium amounts

When you're craving something sweet, creamy, and ooey-gooey, you need to be mindful of the sodium content. Dessert sauces, syrups, and puddings vary in their nature. Most prepared puddings include salt and other sodium-rich foods as ingredients, and many commercially available, fudge-type ice-cream toppings are too high in sodium for a restricted diet. You need to avoid regular pudding mixes, as well, whether preparing the pudding or adding the pudding mix to a recipe.

Hold on to your spoon, though! You can easily prepare decadent, scrumptious puddings and sauces to savor while not wrecking your sodium resolve. You'll be blissfully licking up every last drop of the recipes in this chapter.

Ingredient Safeguards

Many creamy puddings and sauces use milk and other dairy products, as well as eggs, to achieve their rich, silky texture. As long as your recipes are well balanced in their use of these ingredients, the sodium per serving should fit your needs. Watch those recipes heavy in these ingredients.

Chocolate is a favorite flavor when it comes to smooth puddings and sweet sauces. Semisweet chocolate and unsweetened chocolate are good choices for these recipes.

Double-check the amount of milk chocolate called for because this form of chocolate does have some sodium.

Nuts are another favorite addition to sweet sauces. Be sure yours are unsalted.

Watching the Big Dipper

Creamy, rich, and delicious puddings and sauces are very easy to overindulge in. Many times, our eyes are just bigger than our stomachs. To keep your portions in check, you may need to measure out individual servings to be certain you're not getting more than you realize.

If you want a second serving, that's fine, as long as you do it knowingly and tally up the nutrition analysis numbers.

Nutty Chocolate Velvet Sauce

Top your favorite desserts with the delicate crunch of toasted pecans in a buttery chocolate sauce.

Yield:	Prep time:	Cook time:	Serving size:
1¼ cups	5 minutes	10 minutes	2 tablespoons

Each serving has:	
234.9 calories	0 mg sodium

4 TB. unsalted butter	½ tsp. pure vanilla extract
1 cup chopped unsalted pecans	1 cup semisweet chocolate chips

1. In a medium, heavy skillet over medium heat, melt butter. Reduce heat to low, and stir in pecans. Cook, stirring very frequently, for 6 to 8 minutes or until butter is lightly browned and pecans are lightly toasted. Remove from heat.

2. Stir in vanilla extract and chocolate chips until chocolate is melted. Serve warm over frozen yogurt, ice cream, angel food cake, plain pound cake, or white cake, as desired.

Salternative: If you like, substitute chopped unsalted walnuts for the pecans.

Sweet Caramel Sauce

This lightly thickened burnt brown sugar sauce will please your sweet tooth.

Yield:	Prep time:	Cook time:	Serving size:
1 cup	5 minutes	8 minutes	2 tablespoons
Each serving has:			
26 calories	1.4 mg sodium		

1½ TB. firmly packed light brown sugar	1 cup plus 1½ TB. water
1 TB. unsalted butter	1 TB. cornstarch

1. In a small saucepan over high heat, combine light brown sugar, butter, and 1 cup water. Bring to a boil. Remove the saucepan from heat, and reduce heat to medium.

2. In a small cup, whisk together remaining 1½ tablespoons water and cornstarch until blended. Stir into the saucepan, and return to heat. Cook for 5 minutes, stirring occasionally. Remove from heat, and serve hot over ice cream or bread pudding, as desired.

Maple-Walnut Topping

Pure maple syrup sweetens the distinctive crunch of walnuts in this yummy topping.

Yield:	Prep time:	Cook time:	Serving size:
1¾ cups	5 minutes	30 minutes	2 tablespoons
Each serving has:			
130 calories	2.3 mg sodium		

1¼ cups chopped unsalted walnuts	¼ cup water
1 cup pure maple syrup	

1. In a small saucepan over high heat, combine walnuts, maple syrup, and water. Cook until mixture bubbles around the edge of the pan. Reduce heat to low.

2. Cover and cook for 25 minutes or until thickened. Serve hot or cold over ice cream or cake, as desired. Refrigerate leftovers.

Fudge Crackle Coating

Rich and chocolaty, this creamy sauce firms up for a fun coating you can crack into pieces as you eat.

Yield:	Prep time:	Cook time:	Serving size:
2 cups	10 minutes	10 minutes	2 tablespoons
Each serving has:			
195.5 calories	3.9 mg sodium		

1 cup confectioners' sugar

½ cup heavy cream

8 TB. (1 stick) unsalted butter

¾ cup semisweet chocolate chips

4 (1-oz.) squares unsweetened chocolate

1½ tsp. pure vanilla extract

1. In a medium saucepan over medium heat, combine confectioners' sugar, heavy cream, and butter. Cook, stirring constantly, until smooth. (Do not boil.) Remove from heat.

2. Stir in chocolate chips, unsweetened chocolate, and vanilla extract. Stir until chocolate is melted and mixture is smooth. Let cool slightly before serving. Refrigerate any leftovers.

PINCH OF SAGE

Pour this rich sauce over frozen yogurt or ice cream and let it stand until it hardens for a fudgy, cracked coating. You can sprinkle chopped unsalted nuts over the sauce before it sets if you like.

Smooth Chocolate Pudding

The rich taste of chocolate disguises the tofu base of this luscious pudding.

Yield:	Prep time:	Chill time:	Serving size:
2½ cups	10 minutes	1 hour	½ cup
Each serving has:			
325.7 calories	16.7 mg sodium		

1 cup semisweet chocolate chips

2 TB. water

1 (16-oz.) pkg. firm tofu, well
  drained and chopped

¼ cup fat-free milk

1 TB. pure vanilla extract

1. In a small, heavy saucepan over low heat, melt chocolate chips with water, stirring to blend.

2. In a food processor, combine tofu, chocolate mixture, milk, and vanilla extract. Process for 1 or 2 minutes or until blended and smooth, scraping down the sides as necessary. Cover and chill for 1 hour before serving.

PINCH OF SAGE

Don't rush melting the chocolate chips. Keep the saucepan over low heat and melt the chocolate just until you can stir the chips smooth.

Creamy Breakfast Syrup

When you want something other than the ordinary maple syrup, try this sweet and creamy topping with a hint of vanilla.

Yield:	Prep time:	Cook time:	Serving size:
1 cup	5 minutes	10 minutes	2 tablespoons

Each serving has:	
150.6 calories	30 mg sodium

½ cup granulated sugar

½ cup light corn syrup

½ cup light cream

½ tsp. pure vanilla extract

1. In a medium saucepan, combine sugar, light corn syrup, and light cream. Stir to blend, and bring to a boil over medium heat. Boil for 5 minutes or until slightly thickened, stirring occasionally.

2. Remove the saucepan from heat. Stir in vanilla extract. Serve warm over pancakes, waffles, or French toast, as desired.

Cake-Crusted Lemon Pudding

A smooth, tangy-sweet lemon pudding awaits you beneath a crumbly cake topping.

Yield:	Prep time:	Cook time:	Serving size:
2 cups	25 minutes	35 minutes	½ cup

Each serving has:	
246.4 calories	63.9 mg sodium

2 large eggs, separated

1 TB. unsalted butter, softened

2 TB. all-purpose flour

¾ cup granulated sugar

¼ cup fresh lemon juice

1 cup fat-free milk

1. Preheat the oven to 350°F.

2. In a small bowl, and using an electric mixer on medium speed, beat egg whites until frothy. Increase speed to high, and beat until stiff peaks form. Set aside.

3. In a large bowl, and with the mixer on medium speed, beat butter and flour until fine crumbs form. Add sugar, egg yolks, lemon juice, and milk, and beat until well blended. Fold in egg whites.

4. Pour mixture into a pudding dish or a 1-quart baking dish. Bake for 35 minutes or until top is browned. Remove to a wire rack. Serve warm or cold.

PINCH OF SAGE

Make easy work of separating eggs by using an egg separator. Or if you prefer, you can use the tried-and-true method of passing the yolk back and forth from one half of the egg shell to the other. Either way, take care to keep the yolk intact because just a speck of egg yolk in your egg whites will keep them from whipping up.

Creamy Raisin Rice Pudding

The rice-thickened, cinnamon-spiced goodness that is this pudding is studded with sweet raisins.

Yield:	Prep time:	Cook time:	Serving size:
3½ cups	20 minutes	5 minutes	½ cup
Each serving has:			
224.9 calories	65.8 mg sodium		

2 cups uncooked instant white rice

1 (12-oz.) can fat-free evaporated milk

1 cup water

½ cup granulated sugar

½ cup dark raisins

½ tsp. ground cinnamon

1½ tsp. pure vanilla extract

1. In a medium saucepan over high heat, combine rice, evaporated milk, water, sugar, and raisins. Bring to a boil, stirring constantly.

2. Remove the saucepan from heat. Quickly stir in cinnamon and vanilla extract. Cover and let stand for 15 minutes, quickly stirring every 5 minutes. Serve warm or chill to serve cold.

Salternative: If you prefer golden raisins, substitute them in this recipe. Or for a different taste, try any other dried fruit you like—cherries, cranberries, or blueberries.

PINCH OF SAGE

When 60 percent of regular homogenized milk's water is removed, you've got evaporated milk. Evaporated milk and sweetened condensed milk are not interchangeable in recipes. Sweetened condensed milk contains a large amount of added sugar. You can add an equal amount of water to evaporated milk and substitute the mixture for fresh milk in a recipe, which can be more budget friendly, too.

Simply Vanilla Pudding

Delight in pure, unadulterated—and sodium-sensible—vanilla flavor in a spoon-thick, creamy bite.

Yield:	Prep time:	Cook time:	Serving size:
1 cup	5 minutes	15 minutes	½ cup
Each serving has:			
321.7 calories	92.9 mg sodium		

½ cup granulated sugar

2 TB. cornstarch

1½ cups 2 percent milk

1 tsp. pure vanilla extract

1. In a medium saucepan, combine sugar and cornstarch. Gradually whisk in milk.

2. Set over medium heat, and cook, stirring, for 15 minutes or until boiling and very thick. Remove from heat, and stir in vanilla extract.

3. Pour pudding into a small bowl. Cool slightly, and chill for at least 2 hours before serving or until cold.

PINCH OF SAGE

To prevent a thick skin from forming on the top of the pudding, press plastic wrap directly onto the surface of the pudding before chilling.

Wetting Your Whistle

In This Chapter

- Sodium-responsible sippers
- Making healthful beverage choices
- Warm- and cool-weather drinks
- Celebrating with party punches

Reducing the sodium in your diet affects not just your food choices but your beverage consumption as well. Liquid-served sodium counts just as much as food-served sodium or liquid calories—and can be just as overlooked.

Soda, some fruit drinks, even your tap water can add to the sodium intake you're trying to limit. Still, you're unlikely to drink only sodium-free bottled water day in and day out. But don't worry. You can easily prepare flavorful beverages that won't wreck your daily sodium limits. For all the occasions when you want something special to drink, the recipes in this chapter offer a number of tasty options. Cheers!

Punch Bowl Pleasers

We often celebrate special occasions with festive punches and other mingled drinks. But the base ingredients can be sodium-rich sodas, drink mixes, and ice creams.

Whether a wedding, anniversary, baby shower, graduation, bridal shower, or other happy occasion, you, too, can toast its significance while still meeting your low-sodium requirements. You'll want to monitor your number of servings, though. It's easy to keep refilling your cup from the punch bowl that seems never to drain.

Punches made with large amounts of teas, coffees, low-sodium fruit juices, club soda, and sherbets are often good picks. Alternating a punch with other beverages such as black coffee, tea, and bottled water will keep you from feeling deprived while keeping your sodium count in check.

Front-Porch Sippers and Cozy Slurps

Whether you have a front porch or not, the dog days of summer will have you begging for a cold, frosty beverage. The hot-weather classics—old-fashioned lemonade and homemade iced tea—are not only satisfying on a sweltering day, but they're also very low in sodium. Of course, commercial mixes and prepared teas and lemonades may contain sodium; check the nutrition labels.

When you're craving something thicker, try whipping up a smoothie instead of a milkshake. The recipes in this chapter are lower in sodium than what you can get from a fast-food drive-thru and taste great. Or fill a frosty, tall mug with a float, using sodium-free seltzer water instead of the traditional soda. You'll have it made in the shade!

PINCH OF SAGE

If you can't live without soda, you can find a small selection of sodium-free and very low-sodium alternatives.

When the air turns crisp and you just want to curl up inside with a good book, a soothing, hot beverage is in order. But a mug of hot cocoa made with a cup of fat-free milk produces a drink with up to 145 milligrams sodium—and that's not allowing for any marshmallows. The version in this chapter uses nondairy creamer, which is a handy sodium-free alternative.

Tea and coffee are good sodium-free choices. Just be sure you aren't adding too much sodium with your additions. And remember that many flavored tea and coffee mixes do include some sodium; check the labels.

A Cup of Hot Cocoa

With a hint of vanilla, this cup of creamy chocolaty goodness makes you want to curl up in front of a roaring fire.

Yield:	Prep time:	Serving size:
1 cup	5 minutes	1 cup

Each serving has:		
160 calories	3.3 mg sodium	

1 TB. cocoa powder	2 TB. nondairy creamer
2 TB. granulated sugar	¼ tsp. pure vanilla extract
1 cup boiling water	

1. In a mug, combine cocoa powder and sugar. Pour boiling water over top, and stir to dissolve.

2. Stir in nondairy creamer and vanilla extract. Serve immediately.

 SALT PITFALL

If you love to float marshmallows in your cocoa, remember to factor in the additional sodium. You can find the milligrams per serving listed on the nutrition label.

Autumn Spiced Coffee

Transform your black coffee into a creamy, spiced sensation.

Yield:	Prep time:	Serving size:
1 cup	5 minutes	1 cup

Each serving has:		
76.2 calories	5.7 mg sodium	

¼ tsp. plus ⅛ tsp. ground cinnamon

Scant ⅛ tsp. ground cloves

1 cup hot black coffee

1 TB. granulated sugar

1 TB. nondairy creamer

1. In a mug, stir cinnamon and cloves into coffee.

2. Stir in sugar until dissolved. Stir in creamer until blended.

Salternative: Nondairy creamer is a good, sodium-free substitute for real dairy cream. But if you prefer to use cream, just calculate in the bit of sodium it adds, using the information on the nutrition label. You can also adjust the amounts of spices, sugar, and creamer given in this recipe to perfect your personal, pleasurable cup of coffee.

DEFINITION

When a measurement is labeled **scant,** don't overfill the measure. Leave it just a tad short.

Old-Time Lemonade

Enjoy sipping a tall glass of this sweet-tart, front-porch classic on a hot summer afternoon.

Yield:	Prep time:	Serving size:
5 cups	10 minutes	1 cup
Each serving has:		
128 calories	6.2 mg sodium	

4 medium lemons   4 cups water

¾ cup granulated sugar or
   superfine sugar

1. Juice lemons, removing seeds. (You should have about 1 cup lemon juice.) Pour into a pitcher.

2. Stir in sugar, and add water, stirring until sugar is completely dissolved. Chill. Serve in tall glasses over ice.

PINCH OF SAGE

Briefly rolling the lemons on the counter with a little pressure before juicing them yields more juice.

Warm Orange Blossom Tea Punch

Juice-sweetened green tea makes a delicious warming beverage.

Yield:	Prep time:	Cook time:	Serving size:
2 quarts	5 minutes	2 hours, 5 minutes	1 cup

Each serving has:			
102 calories	8.9 mg sodium		

6 cups boiling water	$\frac{1}{3}$ cup granulated sugar
6 individual green tea bags	2 TB. honey
1$\frac{1}{2}$ cups pineapple juice	1 medium navel orange, halved and sliced
1$\frac{1}{2}$ cups unsweetened orange juice	

1. In a large slow cooker, pour boiling water over green tea bags. Let steep for 5 minutes. Discard tea bags.

2. Stir in pineapple juice, orange juice, sugar, and honey. Add orange slices, cover, and cook on low heat for 2 or 3 hours or until heated through and flavors have mingled. Serve warm.

Salternative: You may also chill the slow-cooked punch after it's cooled and serve it over ice, if you prefer.

PINCH OF SAGE

Ladle this pretty punch right from the slow cooker, if you like. After it's heated, the punch will stay hot for some time, so you can turn off the slow cooker.

Splash of Sunshine Punch

Naturally sweet fruit juices pair with the fizz of ginger ale.

Yield:	Prep time:	Chill time:	Serving size:
6½ quarts	5 minutes	1 hour	1 cup
Each serving has:			
119 calories	15.2 mg sodium		

2 qt. apricot nectar

2 qt. pineapple juice

1 qt. unsweetened orange juice

6 cups ginger ale, well chilled

1. In a 2-gallon container, stir together apricot nectar, pineapple juice, and orange juice. Chill for at least 1 hour before serving.

2. Just before serving, pour in ginger ale.

Salternative: You may increase or decrease this recipe as needed.

PINCH OF SAGE

If other large containers are unavailable for mixing, use a clean 1-gallon milk jug.

Old-World Christmas Wassail

Celebrate with this warm mingling of fruit juices, cinnamon, and cloves.

Yield:	Prep time:	Cook time:	Serving size:
3 quarts	5 minutes	10 minutes	1 cup

Each serving has:	
184.6 calories	22.2 mg sodium

2 qt. apple cider	1 cup granulated sugar
2 cups pineapple juice	2 cinnamon sticks
1½ cups unsweetened orange juice	¾ tsp. ground cloves
¾ cup fresh lemon juice	

1. In a large pan over high heat, combine apple cider, pineapple juice, orange juice, lemon juice, sugar, cinnamon sticks, and cloves. Stir. Bring to a boil, and remove from heat.

2. Discard cinnamon sticks, and stir again before serving.

PINCH OF SAGE

If you need to keep this beverage hot during a holiday party, transfer it to a slow cooker set to low heat.

Hot Mulled Cider

This robust apple cider is perfectly flavored with seasonal spices.

Yield:	Prep time:	Cook time:	Serving size:
4 cups	5 minutes	10 minutes	1 cup
Each serving has:			
147.5 calories	27.8 mg sodium		

1 qt. apple cider

2 TB. firmly packed light brown sugar

Pinch nutmeg

4 lemon slices, seeded

8 whole cloves

4 cinnamon sticks

1. In a medium saucepan over high heat, stir together apple cider, light brown sugar, and nutmeg.

2. Stud each lemon slice with 2 cloves, and add cloved lemon slices to the saucepan.

3. Bring mixture to a boil, reduce heat as needed to maintain a simmer, cover, and simmer for 5 minutes. Discard lemon slices.

4. Pour cider into mugs. Garnish each serving with a cinnamon stick.

Salternative: You may double this recipe, if needed. Use a saucepan large enough to hold the mixture comfortably.

Tropical Breeze Smoothie

Yogurt-thickened fruit flavors of pineapple and banana combine in this frothy drink.

Yield:	Prep time:	Serving size:
4 cups	5 minutes	1 cup
Each serving has:		
78 calories	39.8 mg sodium	

1 cup fat-free plain yogurt

¾ cup light lemonade

½ cup crushed pineapple in its
    own juice

1 medium ripe banana, peeled

12 ice cubes

1. In a blender, combine yogurt, lemonade, pineapple, banana, and ice cubes.

2. Blend on high speed for 15 to 20 seconds or until smooth. Serve immediately.

SALT PITFALL

Read nutrition labels carefully. Many yogurts go up in sodium as they go down in fat. We found that our store brand actually fell in sodium as it went from regular to low fat to fat free. The lesson here? Don't dismiss store brands and generics when choosing ingredients.

Frosty Chocolate Raspberry Float

The fizz of seltzer is paired with creamy, cool frozen yogurt in this sweet sipper.

Yield:	Prep time:	Serving size:
2 cups	5 minutes	1 float
Each serving has:		
80 calories	40 mg sodium	

½ cup fat-free vanilla-chocolate
    swirl frozen yogurt

1 cup raspberry-flavored seltzer

1. Scoop frozen yogurt into a tall glass.

2. Pour in seltzer. Serve with a straw and a long-handled spoon.

Salternative: To keep your taste buds happy, try varying the flavors of both the seltzer and the frozen yogurt.

PINCH OF SAGE

Flavored seltzers are a good alternative to soda. You get the fizz of the carbonation without the sodium. You can find these alongside the plain seltzer in the grocery store.

Mocha Latte Punch

Your guests will delight in this smooth, milky coffee with the sweetness of chocolate.

Yield:	Prep time:	Chill time:	Serving size:
1½ quarts	5 minutes	2 hours	½ cup
Each serving has:			
58 calories	52.1 mg sodium		

¼ cup granulated sugar

2 cups strong coffee

6 TB. lite chocolate syrup

4 cups fat-free milk

1. In a large container, stir sugar into coffee until completely dissolved. Stir in lite chocolate syrup, and add milk, stirring until well blended. Chill for at least 2 hours before serving.

2. Stir again before serving. Pour into a punch bowl, and serve over ice.

Salternative: You may increase or decrease this recipe as needed.

SALT PITFALL

Be aware of serving size. This rich punch has a ½ cup serving. If you drink more, be sure to count the additional sodium content.

Coffee-Laced Eggnog Punch

Enjoy a chilled cup of this rich, creamy eggnog mildly coffee flavored.

Yield:	Prep time:	Chill time:	Serving size:
2½ quarts	10 minutes	1 hour	¾ cup
Each serving has:			
179.8 calories	56.9 mg sodium		

½ cup strong coffee

⅓ cup granulated sugar

1 cup hot water

4 cups cold water

1 cup light whipping cream

2 tsp. pure vanilla extract

4 large pasteurized eggs, beaten

1 qt. reduced-fat creamy vanilla ice cream, softened

2 TB. imitation rum extract or to taste

1 tsp. ground nutmeg

1. In a large pitcher, combine coffee, sugar, and hot water, and stir until sugar dissolves. Stir in cold water. Stir in light whipping cream and vanilla extract. Stir in pasteurized eggs. Add ice cream, rum extract, and nutmeg, and stir until ice cream blends into beverage. Chill for at least 1 hour before serving.

2. Stir again before serving. Serve from a chilled punch bowl, and garnish individual servings with an additional sprinkle of nutmeg, if desired.

PINCH OF SAGE

You must use pasteurized eggs in this recipe because the eggs are not cooked. Regular eggs—even if they have clean, uncracked shells—will put you and your guests at risk for illness caused by salmonella bacteria that can cause an intestinal infection.

Banana Bread Smoothie

A touch of almond extract flavors this thick and creamy banana-flavored smoothie.

Yield:	Prep time:	Freeze time:	Serving size:
1½ cups	5 minutes	2 hours	1 smoothie

Each serving has:			
181 calories	102.5 mg sodium		

1 medium ripe banana

3 ice cubes

½ cup fat-free plain yogurt

¼ cup fat-free milk

¼ tsp. pure almond extract

1. Peel and cut banana into 1-inch chunks. Freeze on a small baking sheet or in an empty ice cube tray for 2 hours or until firm.

2. In a blender, combine frozen banana chunks, ice cubes, yogurt, milk, and almond extract. Blend on high speed for 15 to 20 seconds or until smooth and well blended. Serve immediately.

SALT PITFALL

Manufacturers boost milk's taste by adding sodium as they remove fat. The amount of sodium added is minimal, though. Ask your doctor or nutritionist which type of milk is best for you.

Spiced Peach Smoothie

Honey-sweetened, harvest-spiced peaches are thickened with yogurt in this cool drink.

Yield:	Prep time:	Serving size:
1½ cups	5 minutes	1 smoothie

Each serving has:		
271 calories	112.9 mg sodium	

¾ cup frozen peach slices

3 ice cubes

½ cup fat-free plain yogurt

¼ cup fat-free milk

⅛ tsp. ground cinnamon

Dash ground nutmeg

Dash ground allspice

1 tsp. honey

1. In a blender, combine peach slices, ice cubes, yogurt, milk, cinnamon, nutmeg, allspice, and honey.

2. Blend on high speed for 45 to 60 seconds or until smooth and well blended, scraping down the sides as necessary. Serve immediately.

PINCH OF SAGE

Cinnamon is actually the inner bark of a variety of evergreen trees. After the bark is stripped, it's dried in the sun, curling into its recognizable stick form.

Glossary

acini de pepe A small pasta shaped like tiny beads commonly used in soups and cold salads. *See also* pastina.

al dente Italian for "against the teeth." Refers to pasta (or other ingredient, such as rice) that's neither soft nor hard, but just slightly firm against the teeth. This, according to many pasta aficionados, is the perfect way to cook pasta.

allspice Named for its flavor echoes of several spices (cinnamon, cloves, nutmeg), allspice is used in many desserts and in rich marinades and stews.

arugula A spicy-peppery garden plant with leaves that resemble a dandelion and have a distinctive—and very sharp—flavor.

au gratin The quick broiling of a dish before serving to brown the top ingredients. The term is often used as part of a recipe name and implies cheese and a creamy sauce.

balsamic vinegar Vinegar produced primarily in Italy from a specific type of grape and aged in wood barrels. It is heavier, darker, and sweeter than most vinegars.

basil A flavorful, almost sweet, resinous herb delicious with tomatoes and used in all kinds of Italian- or Mediterranean-style dishes.

baste To keep foods moist during cooking by spooning, brushing, or drizzling with a liquid.

Belgian endive A plant that resembles a small, elongated, tightly packed head of romaine lettuce. The thick, crunchy leaves can be broken off and used with dips and spreads.

blanch To place a food in boiling water for about 1 minute (or less) to partially cook the exterior and then submerge in, or rinse with, cool water to halt the cooking.

bouillon Dried essence of stock from chicken, beef, vegetable, or other ingredients. This is a popular starting ingredient for soups because it adds flavor (and often a lot of salt).

bouquet garni A collection of herbs including bay leaf, parsley, thyme, and others traditionally tied in a bunch or packaged in cheesecloth for cooking and subsequent removal.

brine   A highly salted, often seasoned, liquid used to flavor and preserve foods. To brine a food is to soak, or preserve, it by submerging it in brine. The salt in the brine penetrates the fibers of the meat and makes it moist and tender.

broil   To cook in a dry oven under the overhead high-heat element.

broth   *See* stock.

brown   To cook in a skillet, turning, until the food's surface is seared and brown in color, to lock in the juices.

bulgur   A wheat kernel that's been steamed, dried, and crushed and is sold in fine and coarse textures.

caramelize   To cook sugar over low heat until the food develops a sweet caramel flavor. The term is increasingly used to describe cooking vegetables (especially onions) in butter or oil over low heat until they soften, sweeten, and develop a caramel color.

caraway   A distinctive spicy seed used for rye bread as well as pork, cheese, and cabbage dishes. It's known to reduce stomach upset, which is why it's often paired with, for example, sauerkraut.

cardamom   An intense, sweet-smelling spice, common to Indian and Scandinavian cooking, used in baking and coffee.

cayenne   A fiery spice made from (hot) chile peppers, especially the cayenne chile: a slender, red, and very hot pepper.

chickpeas (also **garbanzo beans**)   A yellow-gold, roundish bean that's the base ingredient in hummus. Chickpeas are high in fiber and low in fat, making this a delicious and healthful component of many appetizers and main dishes.

chiles (also **chilis**)   Any one of many different "hot" peppers, ranging in intensity from the relatively mild ancho pepper to the blisteringly hot habañero.

Chinese five-spice powder   A seasoning blend of cinnamon, anise, ginger, fennel, and pepper.

chives   A member of the onion family, chives grow in bunches of long leaves that resemble tall grass or the green tops of onions. Chives provide a light onion flavor to any dish. They're very easy to grow and are often grown in gardens.

cider vinegar   Vinegar produced from apple cider, popular in North America.

cilantro   A member of the parsley family and used in Mexican cooking and some Asian dishes. Cilantro is what gives some salsas their unique flavor. Use in moderation because the flavor can overwhelm. The seed of the cilantro is the spice coriander.

clove   A sweet, strong, almost wintergreen-flavor spice used in baking and with meats such as ham.

coriander   A rich, warm, spicy seed used in all types of recipes, from African to South American, from entrées to desserts.

count   In terms of seafood or other foods that come in small sizes, the number of that item that compose 1 pound. For example, 31 to 40 count shrimp are large appetizer shrimp (often served with cocktail sauce); 51 to 60 count are much smaller.

couscous   Granular semolina (durum wheat) that's cooked and used in many Mediterranean and North African dishes.

cream   To beat a fat such as butter, often with another ingredient such as sugar, to soften and aerate a batter.

cumin   A fiery, smoky-tasting spice popular in Mexican, Middle Eastern, and Indian dishes. Cumin is a seed; ground cumin seed is the most common form of the spice used in cooking.

curing   A method of preserving uncooked foods, usually meats or fish, by either salting and smoking or pickling.

curry   A general term referring to rich, spicy, Indian-style sauces and the dishes prepared with them. A curry will use curry powder as its base seasoning.

curry powder   A ground blend of spices used as a basis for curry and a huge range of other Indian-influenced dishes. All blends are rich and flavorful. Some, such as Vindaloo and Madras, are notably hotter than others. Common ingredients include hot pepper, nutmeg, cumin, cinnamon, pepper, and turmeric. Some curry can also be found in paste form.

custard   A cooked mixture of eggs and milk. Custards are a popular base for desserts.

deglaze   To scrape up the bits of meat and seasoning left in a pan or skillet after cooking. Usually this is done by adding a liquid such as wine or broth and creating a flavorful stock that can be used to create sauces.

devein   To remove the dark vein from the back of a large shrimp with a sharp knife.

dill   A unique herb that's perfect for eggs, salmon, cheese dishes, and, of course, vegetables (pickles!).

dollop   A spoonful of something creamy and thick, such as sour cream or whipped cream.

double boiler   A set of two pots designed to nest together, one inside the other, and provide consistent, moist heat for foods that need delicate treatment. The bottom pot holds water (not quite touching the bottom of the top pot); the top pot holds the ingredient you want to heat.

dredge   To cover a piece of food with a dry substance such as flour or cornmeal.

essential fatty acids   A type of polyunsaturated fat your body obtains from foods, the body being unable to make such fatty acids itself.

fillet   A piece of meat or seafood with the bones removed.

flake   To break into thin sections, as with fish.

floret   The flower or bud end of broccoli or cauliflower.

fold   To combine a dense and light mixture with a circular action from the middle of the bowl.

frittata   A skillet-cooked mixture of eggs and other ingredients that's not stirred but is cooked slowly and then either flipped or finished under the broiler.

fritter   A food such as apples or corn coated or mixed with batter and deep-fried for a crispy, crunchy exterior.

garbanzo beans   *See* chickpeas.

garnish   An embellishment not vital to the dish but added to enhance visual appeal.

grate   To shave into tiny pieces using a sharp rasp or grater.

grind   To reduce a large, hard substance, often a seasoning such as peppercorns, to the consistency of sand.

high-density lipoprotein (HDL)   The type of cholesterol mover that takes cholesterol to the liver to be passed from the body. It's the "good" cholesterol.

hors d'oeuvre   French for "outside of work" (the "work" being the main meal). An hors d'oeuvre can be any dish served as a starter before the meal.

hummus   A thick, Middle Eastern spread made of puréed chickpeas (garbanzo beans), lemon juice, olive oil, garlic, and often tahini (sesame seed paste).

Italian seasoning (also **spaghetti sauce seasoning**)   The ubiquitous grocery store blend of dried herbs that includes basil, oregano, rosemary, and thyme. It's a useful seasoning for quick flavor that evokes the "old country" in sauces, meatballs, soups, and vegetable dishes.

julienne   A French word meaning "to slice into very thin pieces" that are shaped like small matchsticks.

light or **lite**   In reference to sodium, this term labels a product that has less sodium than the regular version, usually 50 percent less.

lite salt   A blend of sodium chloride (salt) and potassium chloride in equal parts.

low sodium   A term used to label foods that contain 140 milligrams or less sodium per serving.

low-density lipoprotein (LDL)   The type of cholesterol mover that can contribute to arterial plaque deposits that can block the arteries. It's the "bad" cholesterol.

marjoram   A sweet herb, a cousin of and similar to oregano, popular in Greek, Spanish, and Italian dishes.

medallion   A small round cut, usually of meat or vegetables such as carrots or cucumbers.

meringue   A mixture of sugar and beaten egg whites, often used as a dessert topping or as cookies when baked, or as a generic ingredient when added to a batter before cooking.

mince   To cut into very small pieces smaller than diced pieces, about $\frac{1}{8}$ inch or smaller.

monosodium glutamate (MSG)   A flavor enhancer that contains about a third the amount of sodium as in table salt.

mull (or **mulled**)   To heat a liquid with the addition of spices and sometimes sweeteners.

nonreactive   A container that is glass, stainless steel, enameled ceramic, or other material that won't react with the acid in a food like aluminum or copper will.

nutmeg   A sweet, fragrant, musky spice used primarily in baking.

oregano   A fragrant, slightly astringent herb used in Greek, Spanish, and Italian dishes.

orzo   A rice-shape pasta used in Greek cooking.

paprika   A rich, red, warm, earthy spice that also lends a rich red color to many dishes.

pastina   A very small pasta, often shaped like stars, beads, rice grains, or alphabet letters.

peppercorns   Large, round, dried berries that are ground to produce pepper.

pesto   A thick spread or sauce made with fresh basil leaves, garlic, olive oil, pine nuts, and Parmesan cheese. Some newer versions are made with other herbs. Pesto can be made at home or purchased and used on anything from appetizers to pasta and other main dishes.

pilaf   A rice dish in which the rice is browned in butter or oil and then cooked in a flavorful liquid such as a broth, often with the addition of meats or vegetables. The rice absorbs the broth, resulting in a savory dish.

pine nuts (also **pignoli** or **piñon**)   Nuts grown on pine trees that are rich (read: high fat), flavorful, and a bit pine-y. Pine nuts are a traditional component of pesto and add a wonderful, hearty crunch to many other recipes.

pita bread   A flat, hollow wheat bread that can be used for sandwiches or sliced, pizza style. Pita bread is terrific soft with dips or baked or broiled as a vehicle for other ingredients.

polenta   Cornmeal mush.

portobello mushrooms   A mature and larger form of the smaller crimini mushrooms, portobellos are brownish, chewy, and flavorful. They're delicious served as whole caps, grilled, and as thin sautéed slices.

presentation   The appealing arrangement of a dish or food on the plate.

purée   To reduce a food to a thick, creamy texture, usually using a blender or food processor.

reduced sodium   A term used to indicate that a food's usual sodium level is reduced by at least 25 percent.

reserve   To hold a specified ingredient for another use later in the recipe.

rice vinegar   Vinegar produced from fermented rice or rice wine, popular in Asian-style dishes. Different from rice wine vinegar.

ricotta   A fresh Italian cheese smoother than cottage cheese with a slightly sweet flavor.

roast   To cook something uncovered in an oven, usually without additional liquid.

rosemary   A pungent, sweet herb used with chicken, pork, fish, and especially lamb. A little rosemary goes a long way.

roux   A mixture of butter or another fat and flour, used to thicken sauces and soups.

saffron   A famous spice made from the stamens of crocus flowers. Saffron lends a dramatic yellow color and distinctive flavor to a dish. Only a tiny amount needs to be used, which is good because saffron is very expensive.

sage   An herb with a musty yet fruity, lemon-rind scent and sunny flavor. It's a terrific addition to many dishes.

salt-free herb and spice seasoning blends   Mixtures of various herbs and spices that are salt-free, MSG-free alternatives to salt.

scant   An ingredient measurement directive not to add any extra, perhaps even leaving the measurement a tad short.

score   A directive to make shallow, incomplete cuts into a food.

Scoville heat scale   A scale used to measure the "hot" in hot peppers. The lower the Scoville units, the more mild the pepper. Ancho peppers, which are mildly hot, are about 1,000 to 2,000 Scovilles; Thai hot peppers are about 50,000 to 100,000; and some of the more daring peppers such as Tears of Fire and habañero are 100,000 to 350,000 Scovilles or more.

separate The process of dividing an egg white from an egg yolk.

sesame oil An oil made from pressing sesame seeds that's tasteless if clear and aromatic and flavorful if brown.

shallot A member of the onion family that grows in a bulb somewhat like garlic and has a milder onion flavor. When a recipe calls for shallot, use the entire bulb. (It might or might not have cloves.)

shellfish A broad range of seafood, including clams, mussels, oysters, crabs, shrimp, and lobster. Some people are allergic to shellfish, so care should be taken with its inclusion in recipes.

shiitake mushrooms Large, dark brown mushrooms originally from the Far East with a hearty, meaty flavor. They can be used fresh or dried, grilled, as a component in other recipes, and as a flavoring source for broth.

simmer To boil gently so the liquid barely bubbles.

skewers Thin wooden or metal sticks, usually about 8 inches long, perfect for assembling kebabs, dipping food pieces into hot sauces, or serving single-bite food items with a bit of panache.

skillet (also **frying pan**) A generally heavy, flat-bottomed metal pan with a handle designed to cook food over heat on a stovetop or campfire.

skim To remove fat or other material from the top of liquid.

sodium An essential mineral the body needs to regulate fluid balance.

sodium free A term used to label foods that contain less than 5 milligrams sodium per serving.

sodium-free baking powder A compound containing no sodium used in place of regular baking powder.

sodium-free baking soda A calcium carbonate product used to replace regular baking soda.

soft-set A stage when eggs have started to firm but aren't yet solid.

steep To let sit in hot water, as in steeping tea in hot water for 10 minutes.

stew To slowly cook pieces of food submerged in a liquid. Also, a dish that has been prepared by this method.

stir-fry To cook small pieces of food in a wok or skillet over high heat, moving and turning the food quickly to cook all sides.

stock A flavorful broth made by cooking meats or vegetables with seasonings until the liquid absorbs these flavors. This liquid is then strained and the solids discarded. Stock can be eaten alone or used as a base for soups, stews, sauces, risotto, or many other recipes.

tamp To tap a pan on a surface to release any air bubbles from a batter.

tarragon A sweet, rich-smelling herb perfect with seafood, vegetables (especially asparagus), chicken, and pork.

thyme A minty, zesty herb whose leaves are used in a wide range of recipes.

tofu A cheeselike substance made from soybeans and soy milk. Flavorful and nutritious, tofu is an important component of foods across the globe, especially from East Asia.

turmeric A spicy, pungent yellow root used in many dishes, especially Indian cuisine, for color and flavor. Turmeric is the source of the brilliant yellow color in many prepared mustards.

very low sodium A term used to label foods that contain 35 milligrams or less sodium per serving.

water chestnuts Actually a tuber, water chestnuts are a popular element in many types of Asian-style cooking. The flesh is white, crunchy, and juicy, and the vegetable holds its texture whether cool or hot.

white mushrooms Ubiquitous button mushrooms. When fresh, they have an earthy smell and an appealing "soft crunch." White mushrooms are delicious raw in salads, marinated, sautéed, and as component ingredients in many recipes.

wild rice Actually a grass with a rich, nutty flavor, popular as an unusual and nutritious side dish.

without added salt A term used to label foods made without the salt that's normally used but may still contain the sodium that's a natural part of the food itself.

yeast Tiny fungi that, when mixed with water, sugar, flour, and heat, release carbon dioxide bubbles, which, in turn, cause the bread to rise. The yeast also provides that wonderful warm, rich smell and flavor.

zest Small slivers of peel, usually from a citrus fruit such as lemon, lime, or orange.

zester A small kitchen tool used to scrape zest off a fruit. A small grater also works well.

Index

Two-Bean Turkey Chili, 94
Wild Turkey Salad, 57
Turkey and Pinto Bean Soft Tacos, 106
Turkey and Swiss in a Green Blanket, 111
Turkey Medallions with Sun-Dried Tomatoes, 206-207
turmeric, 16
Two-Bean Turkey Chili, 94

U–V

unsalted butters, 19
unsalted, defined, 144

vanilla extracts, 18
vegetable side dishes, 283-284
Basil-Tarragon Sautéed Mushrooms, 289
Dilly Carrots Almandine, 299
Green Beans Almandine, 290
Indian-Curried Cauliflower, 298
Oven-Crisped Fries, 285
Quick Cowboy Corn Fritters, 299-300
Roasted Butternut Squash, 293-294
Roasted Potatoes with Basil, 290-291
Splash of Lemon Asparagus, 287
Tomato-Studded Sugar Snap Peas, 295
vegetables, flavorful cooking, 16-18
vegetarian dinners. *See* meatless dinners
Veggie Confetti Frittata, 48
Veggie-Lover's Crunchy Tuna Noodle Casserole, 185

Veggie-Packed Pasta Salad, 55
Veggie-Topped Polenta Pizza Squares, 241-242
Very Berry Tofu Breakfast Smoothie, 28
Vinegar-and-Oil French Dressing, 73
Vinegared Cucumbers, 142
vinegars, 18

W

Walnut-Apricot Dressing, 297
walnuts, 30
Crisp and Creamy Waldorf Dip, 134
Homemaker's Holiday Cranberry Coffeecake, 49
Walnut-Apricot Dressing, 297
Wild Turkey Salad, 57
Walnut-Studded Chocolate Sponge Bars, 325
Warm Orange Blossom Tea Punch, 364
water, sodium content, 5-6
weekends, breakfasts, 37-38
Whole-Wheat Sandwich Flats, 99-100, 254-255
Wild and Brown Rice Pecan Dish, 288
wild rice
Acorn Squash Stuffed with Cranberry-Nut Wild Rice, 243-244
Wild and Brown Rice Pecan Dish, 288
Wild Rice and Berries, 29
Wild Rice and Berries, 29
wild rices, 57
Wild Turkey Salad, 57
Winter Vegetable Spaghetti, 234

X–Y–Z

yeast, 250
Yogurt-Baked Cheesecake, 347

Zesty Vinaigrette Coleslaw, 102, 271
Zippy Jalapeño Hummus, 101, 129
zucchinis
Asian-Flavored Carrot Crunch Salsa, 164
Hearty Grilled Veggie Salad, 56
Pan-Fried Zucchini Rounds, 143